Suffering Insanity

Psychiatric institutions have always been places of fear and awe. Madness impacts on family, friends and relatives, but also on those who provide a caring environment, whether in large institutions of the past, or community care in the present. This book explores the effects of the psychotic patient's suffering on professional carers and the culture of psychiatric services.

Suffering Insanity is arranged as three essays. The first concerns staff stress in psychiatric services, exploring how the impact of madness demands a personal resilience as well as a careful professional support, which may not be forthcoming. The second essay attempts a systematic review of the nature of psychosis and the intolerable psychotic experience, which the patient attempts to evade, and which the carer must confront in the course of daily work. The third essay returns to the impact of psychosis on the psychiatric services, which frequently configure in ways that can have serious and harmful effects on the provision of care. In particular, a service may succumb to an unfortunate schismatic process resulting in sterile conflict, or an assertively scientific culture, which leads to an unwitting depersonalisation of patients.

Suffering Insanity makes a powerful argument for considering care in the psychiatric services as a whole system that includes staff as well as patients; all need attention and understanding in order to deliver care in as humane a way as possible. All those working in the psychiatric services, in both large and small agencies and institutions, will appreciate that closer examination of the actual psychology and interrelations of staff, as well as patients, is essential and urgent.

R.D. Hinshelwood is currently Professor of Psychoanalysis at the Centre for Psychoanalytic Studies, University of Essex. Previously, he was a Consultant Psychotherapist working in mental health services, including the role of Clinical Director of the Cassel Hospital. He is a member of the British Psychoanalytical Society and a fellow of the Royal College of Psychiatrists.

Suffering Insanity

Psychoanalytic essays on psychosis

R.D. Hinshelwood

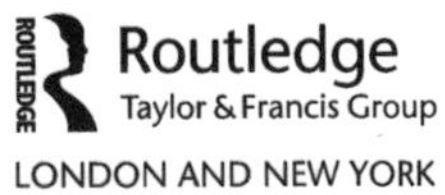

LONDON AND NEW YORK

First published 2004
by Routledge
27 Church Road, Hove, East Sussex BN3 2FA

Simultaneously published in the USA and Canada
by Routledge
270 Madison Avenue, New York NY 10016

Routledge is an imprint of the Taylor & Francis Group, an informa business

Transferred to Digital Printing 2009

Typeset in Times by RefineCatch Limited, Bungay, Suffolk
Paperback cover design by Hybert Design

Paperback cover illustration by Grace Pailthorpe, 16 July 1936, No. 12. 'Five penises at top of head. Two testicles at angle of jaw (reminds me my tonsils were removed at age of 3). I feel my ears straining to be filled this time so the ears must be receptacles. The mouth is to shout with joy and fun.'

This publication has been produced with paper manufactured to strict environmental standards and with pulp derived from sustainable forests.

British Library Cataloguing in Publication Data
A catalogue record for this book is available from the British Library

Library of Congress Cataloging-in-Publication Data
Hinshelwood, R. D.
Suffering insanity : psychoanalytic essays on psychosis / R. D. Hinshelwood.
p. ; cm.
Includes bibliographical references and index.
ISBN 1-58391-893-0 (hardback : alk. paper) – ISBN 1-58391-894-9 (pbk. : alk. paper)
1. Schizophrenia. 2. Countertransference (Psychology) 3. Psychoses. 4. Caregivers.
[DNLM: 1. Schizophrenia—therapy. 2. Schizophrenic Psychology. 3. Caregivers—psychology. 4. Countertransference (Psychology) 5. Professional–Patient Relations. 6. Psychoanalytic Theory.
WM 203 H6645s 2004] I. Title.

RC514.H524 2004
616.89'8–dc22 2004006644

ISBN 978-1-58391-894-4 (pbk)

. . . like a hunk of meat. There was no-one there. He was absent.

(Samuel Beckett 1935)

Contents

Foreword

> Not everything that can be counted counts, and not everything that counts can be counted.
>
> (Albert Einstein)

Practitioners in mental health services and in the Western world are subject to increasing expectations from health authorities, from professional guidelines, from the current zeitgeist for 'evidence'-based approaches and from the increasingly powerfully expressed expectations of users and carers.

In this outstanding series of essays, Bob Hinshelwood takes us 'inside' and 'alongside' those who work with severe mental disturbance. In his Introduction he emphasises that he is writing this book in order to illustrate as fully as possible the *psychological* impact and responses of professionals to their mentally ill patients who cannot cope at a particular point with aspects of life. He wants this book to balance the many treatises on *medical* responses to such people, which tend to downplay the subjective, which leads to the psychology of the mental health professions and psychiatrists becoming neglected.

He illustrates, with admirable clarity, that it is in fact the nature of these ubiquitous *psychological* responses in individuals and groups of professionals that will play a central role in determining whether the expectations just referred to have some chance of being fulfilled, and in determining the quality of the service provided. He does this in a way that does not diminish the importance of biological and medical approaches, but his aim is clearly to get a better balance, to provide better bridges between models and between patients and practitioners and services and to describe everyday crucial psychological phenomena that have never been, and perhaps never could be, subject to evidence-based medicine approaches.

Amongst some of the core issues he highlights are the facts that, for whatever reason, people with mental illness have disturbances in their identity, a loss or altered meaningfulness of their lives and relationships, and have lost control of aspects of themselves and their capacities to use their minds to negotiate their life journey and its hazards. This is common knowledge. What is not adequately recognised is that clinical contact brings these very issues right into the minds of the practitioner and arouses potentially disturbing or enabling psychologically determined subjective responses. These responses can often unwittingly parallel those of the patients, e.g. perpetuating the meaninglessness and loss of identity, excessive and prolonged taking over of control and creating an excessive distance or disconnection from the disturbing life issues. They lie behind the phenomenon of institutionalisation that can refer just as much to community approaches as to those in asylums. The book has a number of very clear examples.

The phenomena Bob Hinshelwood refers to are not commonly discussed but are easily observed, and it is not too difficult to conduct formal research to demonstrate their existence. The same research can at the same time provide clear evidence that current psychiatric training does not usually equip psychiatrists with the skills to address these problems at an interpersonal level (McCabe *et al.* 2002). Nevertheless it is these very psychological responses and how they are managed that are crucial determinants of the outcome for both patient and practitioner and to the way in which services are organised and focused.

There is currently a healthy indignation at much of the way in which psychiatric practice is and has been practised. A good deal of this indignation comes from within psychiatry (McGorry 2000) and psychology (Bentall 2003; BPS 2001). This indignation is well intentioned but runs the risk of being unhelpfully attacking, arousing defensive responses that do not move the situation on.

Speaking personally, in my own work in west London, where Bob Hinshelwood himself worked for many years, I have been greatly inspired by the practices and attitudes of a number of Scandinavian colleagues and groups, who seem to be able to better maintain their 'equilibrium' and a 'mindful' interest in their patients in the face of psychosis and adopt a less reductionistic approach. These colleagues have been prominent contributors to the increasingly worldwide network known as the ISPS (the International Society for the Psychological Treatments of Schizophrenia and other Psychoses).[1]

Through this book Bob Hinshelwood makes a very substantial contribution to this approach, which enhances the possibilities of working with people with psychosis in a more 'mindful' way; he does this paradoxically by focusing in a sophisticated manner on those very psychological processes that can render us relatively mindless when faced with psychosis. In the sense that his book takes the raw everyday observable phenomena of patient–clinician encounters, Bob is truly reporting a particular form of science. After describing the phenomena in Chapter 1, he moves onto explaining the phenomena within a theoretical framework in Chapter 2. In the final essay in Chapter 3, he gives a very rich description of how the phenomena and the theoretical underpinning can be used within services to better attend to the staff who are 'suffering insanity' and gradually assist their patients and clients to be able to manage their suffering more.

The book is a very timely one in that there is now widespread recognition (UKCC 1998) that, in many settings in both wards and community mental health centres, there has been an erosion of time that used to be regularly set aside for staff or staff and patients to reflect on how the setting was functioning. As this time is reclaimed, managers of mental health services and team leaders need to have clear ideas and concepts and skills involved in optimising what is now often called the 'reflective space'.

The phenomena that the book refers to will always be present in those spaces whether attended to or not. Bob Hinshelwood has given us a chance to look and think again as to how we tend to deal with the phenomena. His book is therefore a wonderful opportunity to reflect on how we can minimise the chances of institutionalisation and depersonalisation of care as we develop new services for patients and try to offer the optimum in our current services. The book will be invaluable to all mental health practitioners, leaders of mental health teams and those responsible for commissioning services and leading their implementation. I am convinced that this book will become a classic and will therefore long remain a

1 For information about the ISPS see: www.isps.org

standard recommendation for reading and re-reading as a guide and inspiration to reflection on our everyday practice.

Brian Martindale

Brian Martindale is Consultant Psychiatrist in Psychotherapy, West London Mental Health Trust, Chair of ISPS UK (UK branch of International Society for the Psychological Treatments of Schizophrenia and other Psychoses), Western European Zone representative of the World Psychiatric Association, and Honorary President of the European Federation of Psychoanalytic Psychotherapy in the Public Sector.

References

Bentall, R.P. (2003) *Madness Explained. Psychosis and Human Nature*. London: Penguin.

British Psychological Society (BPS) (2001) Recent advances in understanding mental illness and psychotic experiences. Report by the British Psychological Society Division of Clinical Psychology, London.

McCabe II., R., Heath, C., Burns, T., and Priebe, S. (2002) Engagement of patients with psychosis in the consultation: conversation analytic study. *British Medical Journal* 325: 1148–1151.

McGorry, P.D. (2000) The scope for preventive strategies in early psychosis: logic, evidence and momentum. In M. Birchwood, D. Fowler and C. Jackson (eds) *Early Interventions in Psychosis*. Chichester: John Wiley.

United Kingdom Central Council (UKCC) for Nursing, Midwifery and Health Visiting Disabilities Nursing (1998) Reflective practice – a guide to working with vulnerable clients. London: UKCC.

Acknowledgements

The enjoyment of writing this book has been to recall all those people who helped me learn my psychiatry, patients especially, as well as colleagues. I owe a great deal to the many colleagues in psychiatry I worked with, especially during my 17 years at St Bernard's Hospital in West London, during the great reorganisation towards community care. But I owe a particular impetus for writing this down to Mario Perini and the course 'Helping to help', which he invited me to teach. As Consultant Psychotherapist for over 20 years in the Psychiatric Service of the NHS, I have many colleagues whom I have learned from and debated with. I think of Jack Steinert, and Colin McEvedy who tolerated my psychoanalytic ways, and other psychoanalysts: Dennis Brown, Richard Carvalho, Alicia Etchegoyen, David Riley, Harold Bourne, Bernard Baruch, Dave Bell and Wilhelm Skogstad. I have valued the unending discussion with Hebe Comerford about the way the NHS culture changes. Nothing is ever a personal achievement, only a group process.

Introduction

I imagine everyone has had some life experience that creates the reaction, 'I can't cope with this'. What this means when one has no alternative but to deal with the experience probably has very individual significance to each one of us. It may be slumping into a chair with the bank manager's letter in your hand, or getting on the phone immediately to your sister with the news that mother has just died, or going to the pub instead of back home to the wife after you've just been given the sack. These are things you do . . . but what does it feel like? It can be almost impossible to capture in words, and perhaps the closer to the extreme, the less possible it is to express articulately – expletives, tears and physical actions have to substitute.

After my father died, I can recall going to see him in the chapel of rest. On seeing him, I did not see 'his body'. I saw *him*. To my mind he was about to sit up and say, 'hallo, Bob'. There was a kind of confrontation inside me between the actual dead body, and the real man, the person, my father. I could have said to myself, which of those is most real – the body or the father? But at the time all I could think was that the body would rise up and greet me, exactly as he would have done a week before. It was a moment of real encounter with him. My experience was a devastating one, and I recall the only thing in my mind was to clutch physically at something. The nearest thing was my wife's hand. I suppose I felt like falling down. Later she told me I held her hand so hard it was very painful, and she had wanted to pull away. It was a bodily feeling, something right through my body, as if it were full to bursting with something, not exactly physical pain. It felt more like emptiness, bursting with emptiness, all over. I do not have much confidence that this can mean a lot to the reader, who must supply his or her own extreme experience to fill in the description here. Indeed, is it possible to capture such a sense that something is happening to you that will only damage or destroy you?

Now what if you take your own worst experience of this kind, and double it, or multiply ten-fold? What if you have no-one to clutch onto, no-one at all? Is that anything like the experience a psychotic patient has? Can we know if it is? I don't know if I can consciously have anything like the psychotic experience, or if it matches anything I have known consciously. I can only try to picture my worst experience. Perhaps the schizophrenic is endowed in some neurological way to have a 'worst experience' very frequently when he encounters real events. Maybe, too, he has been subject to a life that teaches him there is no-one he can clutch onto.

This book is about the psychotic experience as it figures within the frame of professional care. It shares my puzzled efforts to make some sense of that experience with others who are struggling too. In this sense, I am writing a certain kind of psychology: the psychology of carers, of professional carers, and especially carers in mental illnesses. I want to create something that will balance those textbooks and journals that concentrate on the medical treatment of psychotic people.

Therefore, this is about the dark side of experience. It is not a happy book. It is about the struggle with psychic pain of the most extreme sort. Facing such experience requires some fortitude, which all psychiatric carers have. But for all of us it has a cost. Psychosis impacts on us.

For many centuries, probably since the human race began, there have been ways of making sense of madness. Caring for psychotic people[1] demands a way of thinking about it, and explaining it. Psychosis has also required special social institutions in which the experience can be contained. From medieval times, psychotic people were cared for in religious institutions, where it was believed that alien demons invaded the victims' minds. The medicalisation of the care of the psychotic from the late eighteenth century may at times have been more humane, but it came with a new set of assumptions: that the mind of the psychotic is in process of irrevocable disintegra-

1 I concentrate on schizophrenia as there is a relative neglect of psychoanalytic studies of the other major psychosis, manic-depressive illness, although it has attracted some attention (Abraham 1911, 1924; Freud 1917a; Meltzer 1963; Jackson 1993; Rey 1994; Lucas 1998). In fact the use of the term 'psychosis' in this book is synonymous with schizophrenia.

tion. The best that could be done would be to delay the process; and the treatment was incarceration in an asylum. This intense pessimism lifted around the turn of the twentieth century, not least because of the expansion of psychological methods, including psychoanalysis. Although psychoanalysis contributed to the optimism of the 'new psychiatry' at the turn of the twentieth century, at first it remained pessimistic about psychosis. The torch of optimism was enthusiastically taken up in the late twentieth century by biological psychiatry and the pharmaceutical advances in brain-active drugs. Nevertheless, the role of psychoanalysis has not shrunk to zero. Potentially it has an intensely important role. Even if that role is not in terms of direct cure, it informs us about the caring relation in psychiatry.

The late twentieth century saw another turn within psychiatry, i.e. the integration of psychiatric care into the general community. Community care is part of the current optimism, but it is also suspect. It may be that we have drawn not only patients into the community, but also a lot of the psychological and institutional problems from the old hospitals. When I worked in the late 1960s in the first day hospital in this country (the Marlborough Day Hospital was founded in 1948) I found myself, with the rest of the staff, fumbling to manage the boundary between institutional care and community care. There were psychodynamic processes around the forming of the day hospital every morning and the relinquishing of the patients to their community in the evening that bewildered us, and told us that de-institutionalisation had to be closely studied (see Hinshelwood 1987a, 1994a). For community care to succeed, there needs to be a sensible awareness of why the medicalised mental hospitals did their job so badly. If we really wish to avoid dragging the same problems into the community, we need to gauge the full impact of psychosis on the community carers, in a way that we never properly did in the old hospitals (Hinshelwood 2001).

Despite the arduous nature of the experience I deal with, this book is intended to be a resource for those working in the psychiatric services, in both large and small agencies and institutions. All staff who have a 'hands-on' aspect to their work need to reflect on the fact that they too 'suffer' insanity, as well as their patients. Indeed, it could be said that they frequently do so instead of their patients. This will therefore be a text for teaching in nursing and medical schools, as well as other paramedical trainings. It is intended more for professional carers, but families too may gain something of an understanding of how our psychiatric services attempt to help, and our limits. I have not wanted to write a teaching text on how to employ a psychoanalytic method or make interpretations. Instead, I have sought to expand awareness of the relational and emotional nature of psychiatric care, without flinching. It takes its place among various recent psychodynamically oriented works, such as the Cassel Monograph Series (Griffiths and Pringle 1997; Day and Pringle 2001) and *Face to Face with Distress* (Barnes *et al.* 1998), which aim to present a particular approach to the 'use of the self'. Ellwood (1995) and Berke *et al.* (2001) also describe particular attempts to relate to psychosis, rather than merely to treat it. Williams (2001) provides a varied, though not systematic, selection of psychoanalytic reflections on psychosis.

In the first essay, the impact that psychosis has on the personal experience of carers is explored, along with various means that people take to minimise that impact. I wanted to highlight the importance of the disorders of meaning and identity that afflict schizophrenic patients, because they contaminate psychiatric workers with similar afflictions. Meaninglessness and identity-distortions are occupational hazards, but not much in the way of occupational health measures is deployed in our services to cope with those hazards. I give weight to the particular support that is required, as a matter of course, to deal with the personal impact. I describe how support needs to be reality-oriented and focused on levels of achievement by the staff.

Essay 2, in a different gear, becomes more theoretical. Although psychoanalysis has not proved to be a treatment of individual patients suffering from psychosis, there is a huge amount of psychoanalytic description of patients' experiences. This is a major resource as a way into the extreme experiences we encounter in the day-to-day work. This body of literature is also a major attempt to give an articulate, coherent and meaningful account of the experience. Much of this is in the arcane terminology of the various psychoanalytic schools. The gulf between the formulated theory and the original experiences with patients is often huge, and unbridgeable for all but those within the 'holy circle'. The essay attempts, insofar as it has been possible for me, to give some stepping-stones to traverse this gulf. I use a published account of a psychoanalytic assessment interview with a severe long-standing schizophrenic patient, in order to try to give some flesh and blood to the theoretical skeleton. To the degree that I have made psychoanalytic theorising of psychosis accessible, it brings a little meaning to what is meaningless, and hence a degree of support against the impact of psychotic meaninglessness.

The third and last essay returns to the impact of psychosis as it is transmitted through the individual carers into the service, agencies and institutions of psychiatry. I have tried over many years to point to the institutional effects and disorders that result (e.g. Hinshelwood 1979, 1987b, 2001). I try to capture this social pathology in terms of distortions of our task, and schisms within our teams, agencies and social groupings. All these institutional effects arise from, and in turn reflect back upon, our sense of identity as psychiatric carers.

Finally, the epilogue puts together the struggle that psychotic patients face in overcoming an alienation of self, on one hand, and the more normal 'healthy regression', as it is called, on the other. The psychotic problems are overwhelmingly greater, but some first steps can be mapped out as a guide to what might be accomplished in a complementary way to the physical methods of treatment. The task, in short, is to help the psychotic rather than his carers to suffer his psychosis more fully.

Essay 1

Helping to help

The impact of madness on those who care

> Schizophrenia is an expertise in producing disquiet in others.
> (Berke 1979, p. 23)

All work makes us stressed, the simplest because of its tedium, the most difficult because of its responsibility. Some work is both tedious and responsible. The most stress comes when the work involves caring for other people – i.e. being responsible for others. Responsibility for other people is the greatest responsibility felt by humans.

Perhaps responsibility is a biological inheritance, due to becoming a social species. It has a central significance in human psychology. Responsibility for others is our foundation as ethical animals. Generally speaking, care work is that of the professions: pastoral, medical, nursing, educational. The professions entail work that is carried out on and for others, as persons. They contrast with the work of those who make cars, or who look at stars through a telescope, or whose main concern is the bottom-line of profit or loss on a sheet of accounts.[1]

Schizophrenia has the effect of corrupting that responsibility. Our identity as professional carers becomes disquietingly merged with that of our patients, and, in another direction, our identity becomes unrealistically separate. I shall explore this problem of responsibility and the identity of carers in psychiatry in this first essay.

1 Of course, the balance of accounts is important. However, rhetoric in Western societies risks elevating financial balances above all other values. In fact, I would argue (though not here) that humans actually value their responsibility to and for each other more highly. The monetarist rhetoric renders those more personal values inappropriately quiet in the historical present.

There are two major features to the experience of schizophrenia. One is responsibility and identity; the other is meaninglessness and understanding. In schizophrenia, the world loses meaning, and in place of that loss a patient reconstructs a new meaning. However, the new meaning comes out of his imagination to form convincing delusions and hallucinations, which populate his world in place of a true interest in the world we all live in. This means that the capacity to understand things in real ways and with reflective thought is hampered in the condition, and that spreads to those who care for schizophrenics. Understanding is the second core feature in the experience of psychosis and in the experience of caring for it.

These two areas – (a) responsibility and identity, and (b) meaninglessness and understanding – are not just key to the psychotic condition, but key areas in a psychology of care as well. That is to say, certain things specifically about schizophrenia have an impact on specific issues in the psychology of those who care for schizophrenics. In particular, the corruption of responsibility affects the identity of carers; and the meaninglessness of the schizophrenic's world gives a priority to finding meaning and 'understanding': an understanding either of the condition or of the experience.

The psychology of care

The work of care is most arduous because of the psychological dimension, and that dimension results in the most stress (some 13.5 million hours per year are lost due to stress in the NHS, out of a workforce of around one million). The raw material of the work is other human beings. Therefore we have a human relationship with the work itself, so it is not ordinary work. It is emotional, and it involves us in personal ways as people. That sets caring apart. Also for that reason, it can acquire an elite status. Perhaps the most responsible work of all is caring for those with severe psychological difficulties. Because we are human beings, we must supplement the ordinary psychology of work, job satisfaction, morale, financial motivation, and so forth, with the psychology of human relations. Added to that, in psychiatry the human relations side of the work is a lot more difficult since the work is with particularly difficult people. We may frequently have to accept non-compliance with treatment and the misinterpretation of our good intentions. Because patients may be delusional and frightened, our role of carer may not be confirmed by those we care for.

We may not in the past have paid as much attention to the psychology of people who care for the mentally ill as they deserve, or need. There are certain reasons why this kind of work study has been neglected. The strongest of those reasons is that we look after not just humans but the irrational human, and irrationality of the most extreme kind.[2] Attitudes to rationality have been strengthened, and the emotive and irrational side of human beings has been progressively submerged into an unattended nether region. It may therefore be that psychiatric services are increasingly at variance with the encroaching ethos of Western institutions of all kinds. If we want to increase the scope of the psychology of work, then in psychiatry particularly we should turn to a psychology of the irrational. There are various kinds of psychology, and they do not all address the irrational. In this book, I use psychoanalysis because it does not place rationality at a higher level than irrationality. It does not simply say that the irrational is abnormal. To regard it as abnormal is irrational. Psychoanalysis can sometimes explain our irrationality about things, and can explain how we can react irrationally to irrationality.

Moreover, where attention has been paid to the psychology of mental health work, the most useful interventions may not have been adequately thought through. So, supporting the teams of staff may not have been effective. Supportive interventions need to take account of both the rationality *and the irrationality* in the working system.

The impact of psychosis

Psychiatric services are now more or less psychosis services. The concentration of psychotic people all together creates a rather specific kind of institution, one that is emotionally frightening. In such an institution, two 'kinds' of people, patients and staff, identify themselves as strictly one or the other. Often it is a negative identity – staff are *not* patients, for example. Group identity is then very strong, and staff and patients influence each other on this stereotyped basis (these phenomena will be discussed further in Essay 3). Staff aim to exert a beneficial influence: to aid patients to recover, and resume

2 It may be unfortunate for the psychiatric services that, while over recent decades the ethos of managing people has crept in, it has been a style of management that has been called rational management, or scientific management (see Essay 3).

whatever level of life they can manage. But it does not work out so simply. We know the influence may not be beneficial. Unhealthy dependency and institutionalisation can afflict the patients, but there is also a reverse direction to the influence: patients affect staff. Sometimes they affect staff beneficially when patients recover and express gratitude, thus giving the staff an implicit emotional support. However, that kind of beneficial influence is often in short supply in psychiatry. Frequently, recovery is only partial, and gratitude is often numbed by the patients' maladaptive relationships. So patients' influence on staff can be detrimental.

The psychological states of staff and patients interact. This is called 'parallel process', a term introduced by Stanton and Schwartz (1954). They meant that something happening on the staff side of the institution would be reflected in the patient community. They were concerned particularly with emotional states that spread from one side of the institution to affect the emotional states on the other side. They observed that at a time of high levels of staff anxiety about financial survival, a larger number of patients were transferred to the secure ward. This kind of transport of anxiety occurred without intention and probably unconsciously. The opposite also happens, from patients to staff. That transmission is largely what we will discuss. The following, from when I was a young psychiatrist, was an individual interview:

> A young woman came to the outpatient clinic. She had previously been in hospital for a number of months and, typical of a chronic schizophrenic person, she had little affect or initiative. Each time I saw her I found myself trying to instil some hope and enthusiasm into her – to think of a job, to make friends, to attend a psychiatric social club. Each time she agreed with me . . . and I felt better. Each time she came back to the next appointment, she had done nothing. I would feel despondent and set about renewing my efforts to enthuse her.

She came with her overwhelming despairing, and in the course of the contact I too became despairing. This could be repeated endlessly. In this case, a non-cognitive communication was exchanged between us. The upshot was my need to relieve *my* despair. She allowed that to happen, rather than making any real effort to improve her own life.

The process was that despair was transported from one person to another. We normally expect others to communicate with us through words, but in this case the primary communication was not exactly in words. She did not say 'I am despairing'. Of course, ordinary relationships, too, are based on much more than words. In fact a certain kind of direct effect on another person's emotions is especially effective in supplementing words. We might think of the cries of a baby, which affect mother very deeply without any clear semantic meaning or symbolic content to the noise. This is common in psychiatry, too. Hidden and often unwitting (unconscious) communications occur with great impact. In my example, the communication first of all was that the patient's despair became my despair. In turn, the patient received from me a communication that I was despairing and needed her acquiescence to relieve me – which she loyally did. This was a completely different set of communications from the ones I thought we were making. Consciously, I thought I was giving her good ideas that met her need. I thought I enthused her with hope. Unconsciously, though, I clearly indicated my despair, and what I needed from her; and she picked up that unwitting communication.

A similarly complex transaction is the giving and taking of drugs. It involves a set of conscious communications. However, running beside them are other, and unconscious, communications frequently transacting something quite different. Sometimes we give drugs because we don't know what to do, and it averts a feeling of impotence; or they help us avoid talking to patients and thereby keep us emotionally distant from psychotic people. Even psychotic patients can be attuned to such implicit messages.

We need to emphasise to ourselves, and to each other, these important conclusions when we work with psychotic people:

- they do affect their helpers;
- those effects are emotionally unpleasant;
- the effects may be communicated unconsciously;
- our actions may be unwittingly motivated to ease these communications for ourselves.

Whether we accept or are aware of it, an interactive psychological process is almost certainly taking place between us and even the most psychotic patient. This must be a beginning to a psychology of care.

Responsibility and professional identity

If we peer through a magnifying glass at the emotional currents during the admission of a patient to a psychiatric ward, we will see a complex turbulence. The following is a description of a psychotic patient who caused worry about herself with her outrageous behaviour, as effective as if she had removed her clothes and walked along Piccadilly in the middle of the road against the flow of traffic (Conran 1985, p. 40).

> The feelings induced in the doctor and nurses were of the woman's wildness and unpredictability and that they were called upon to manage her, to control her and, above all, to stop the incessant flow of unintelligible chatter. In common parlance, they felt called upon to *'shut her up'* . . . We may note that whatever the anxieties and opinions of those outside the hospital, these had now to find resolution within the hospital . . . the patient does not suffer her pain, rather as intolerable anxiety, of being bereft of self-control, it is projected into the hospital staff who are engaged to suffer it for her. The staff then deal with it . . . as best they are able, generally altogether ignorant as to the sources of the patient's anxiety – indeed, they scarcely even recognise it as anxiety. (Conran 1985, p. 37)

The staff and the hospital had come to have charge of a patient who was no longer able to control or care for herself. So, having charge of her meant a fairly extensive burden of care. That care was literally to make up for the patient's lack of self-control, and self-care.

This transmission, effected without words, is a radical communication. The patient lost her self-care function and it was transported, to all intents and purposes, to the caring staff. Moreover, this is not the care of a patient as in a general hospital, where there may be a need to care for the patient's helpless body, even an unconscious patient's body. In this instance it is the patient's personality. It is the capacity to be a person that she has lost and the staff somehow have to find for themselves. A heavy onus falls on the staff in admissions of this kind. They must accept the government of the whole person.

This is often a thankless task. When a patient has dismantled the capacity to be responsible for himself, he has lost the capacity to know that staff are doing a good job for him. Staff must cope with little or no appreciation from the patient. We need appreciation from clients like all other professionals, but psychiatric staff are denied reliable support of that kind. Problems of job satisfaction crop up for professionals who work with clients who cannot properly express the value of the worker. Like everyone, we need the work to reflect back our skills and our achievements, but psychiatric staff have to face uncertain outcomes and successes with patients who may never feel grateful. Carers have to suffer the consequences of the responsibility they have and also that which is unnaturally placed upon them.

Institutionalisation

Staff who are responsible for patients' decisions, for self-care and for the very meaning of their lives, can come to institutionalise this state of affairs. That is to say, they institutionalise a psychological state of affairs. In that state they are solely the responsible ones, and their patients are not responsible for their own decisions:

> only roles of health or illness are on offer; staff to be only healthy, knowledgeable, kind, powerful and active, and patients to be only ill, suffering, ignorant, passive, obedient and grateful. (Main 1975, p. 61)

A division comes down between patients and staff, in which patients become stereotyped; and of course staff become stereotypes of a complementary kind. Patients end up suffering more from the institution than from the illness. As David Clark commented about the old psychiatric institutions, the chronic schizophrenic 'was the result, not of his schizophrenia, but of the way he had been "looked after" for several decades' (Clark 1964, p. 14). This pernicious process is particularly connected with a specific disorder of schizophrenia. The patient has off-loaded his responsibility, in the most drastic but typical way. And the staff are obliged, and willing, to accept the divergent roles of patient and staff. By creating the stereotype of a patient, he becomes a different species of human. Staff treat such people accordingly, more as children, or as difficult children. *One Flew over the Cuckoo's Nest* (Kesey 1962) was a painful likeness of that numbing obliteration of respectful human relations.

The separation between the perception of healthy staff and unhealthy patients has been well attested. It is interpreted in various ways: as power relations (Goffman 1961; Foucault 1967), as political relations (Laing 1967, Scull 1977), as a treatment relation (Main

1975, Rosenberg 1970), or as real and rational as in scientific, diagnostic psychiatry (e.g. the DSM; American Psychiatric Association 1994), and so on. Whatever the explanation, the stereotype is a cumbersome piece of baggage. And it is self-contradictory in that if staff really were so healthy and wise, they would not feel, and be, so endlessly in difficulties; in addition, the need for patients to be helplessly ill must militate against allowing them to grow and heal.

Tom Main, writing primarily of doctors, says that:

> the medical man, educated to play a grandiose role among the sick, finds it difficult to renounce his power and shoulder social responsibilities in a hospital and to grant sincerely to his patients independence and adulthood. But it is no easier for the rest of the staff. (Main 1946, p. 10)

The reality that the staff are themselves vulnerable, too, and they can feel disturbed, needs to be grasped, though we must balance that recognition with the reality that staff are not highly vulnerable, and are not as vulnerable as psychotic patients.

There is a motivated 'stuckness' about this institutionalised set of roles and professional identities. This is in part to do with the particular kind of care the psychotic patient requires, and with the vulnerability of the staff. The quality of concern and care that a schizophrenic patient asks is quite out of the ordinary. It goes beyond normal professional care, and has implications for the outcome of the care. In the instance of a physical illness, such as an appendicitis, the patient once physically recovering can psychologically recover too, and he 'resumes the governance of himself' (see Conran's (1985) comparison of a psychotic woman with a surgical case of appendicitis, and also the epilogue). However, the resumption of self-governance and self-determination can be hindered, and that can occur in mental hospitals and with psychotic patients. In that situation, patients may not properly resume responsibility for themselves and we as staff go on 'being' their responsibility. Especially in the mental health sphere, staff may frequently have to know best, even though in contemporary medicine we are moving away from this paternalistic position to one where the patient is expected to know what is wrong and to choose her own treatment in an act of consent. It is not of course certain how much patients want to make, or psychologically can make, decisions when in severe pain, stressed or frightened. So informed consent is an ideal, officially required, but with human frailty it is not always attainable. When it comes to psychiatry there is a very pressured situation for staff to take on an extreme responsibility – responsibility for the actual person, not just his body. Very often psychotic patients are hardly recognisable as people. After a visit to a mental hospital, Samuel Beckett described a particular schizophrenic patient as a 'hunk of meat' (quoted in Knowlson 1996, p. 209).

Meaninglessness and understanding

This lump-of-meat quality arises largely because of the different worlds that patients live in, worlds that barely overlap with the world of the staff or ordinary people. It arises from the lack of shared meaning between patients and staff; indeed, it may even be the loss of meaning altogether in the schizophrenic's world.

It is important for staff to have a meaning to their job, and what they do for their patients. Barrett (1996) approached this problem as an anthropologist. He showed how the 'meaningless' state of a schizophrenic on admission is processed in different ways at different stages, to bring the patient back towards an ordinary human condition. This 'anthropology of psychiatry' was elucidated as follows.

Anthropologists visit other cultures to record their myths and social systems. They try to understand how other people make sense of their own worlds, and what principles they use for giving meaning to the world and to their experiences. What does it mean that the sun rises each day, in a certain place on the horizon, and so on? What does it mean to feel bereaved, to lose someone, who no longer exists? There is an infinite variety of ways of making sense of these life experiences. To a degree the philosophy of life depends on what sort of place the people live in – if it is by the sea then their myths and meanings have to do with the sea and its fruits and dangers. In a crowded metropolitan environment, myths have to do with the busy bustle, cramped space and ambitions that mark out such places. Barrett observed a psychiatric ward in this way, anthropologically. What meaning did the staff give the patients' behaviour, utterances, hallucinations and delusions, and so on? He recorded the characteristic 'rituals' that seemed to be repeated there. The psychiatric ward is perhaps special, because its rituals do not reiterate cultural meanings; rather, meaning is made out of something meaningless.

The admission of a patient is made sense of in phases, something like this (my description, though based on Barrett's observations):

> Initial examination on admission reveals the illness, schizophrenia. It is some 'thing' that happens to the patient. It removes their personhood because what happens to them is viewed as the illness, not as them. The patient is conceived as symptoms, bits that can be put together as a syndrome. The person of the patient is a set of static characteristics that has, as it were, taken him over. That is the occurrence that has happened to him.
>
> The next stage, as Barrett describes it, is the 'worked-up case'. The psychiatric team pool all their knowledge of the patient and make a narrative of the triggers and processes of the incipient illness. They elaborate a coherent picture of the fully-fledged acute psychotic state beneath which the person has submerged, and they make a prognosis or prediction of how he will turn out. A full narrative of the disease process has been reconstructed from the disparate pieces of knowledge gathered by the team. An integration process in the form of a narrative has begun. Treatment of a biological kind is then instituted to control the causation of the illness.
>
> Thereafter, as things improve, in the final stage the patient begins to emerge from the helpless dominance of his symptoms, and can bring back his own self-determination. His state is no longer illness-determined. In other words, he is reinstated as a person, a moral being who can make his own decisions. (after Barrett 1996)

The trajectory is from acute psychosis to a reconstructed whole person; it is a process of 'taking apart and putting back together again' (Barrett 1996, p. 268). In the course of the journey through these standard stages, the psychiatric team conducts various procedures which in anthropological terms look like rituals. These give a standard meaning to the object of study at each phase, which is supplementary to any biological or pharmacological effect. This process, when it goes well, makes a meaningful sense of the schizophrenic condition, and it is staff that need it. Staff need to feel meaning in their work. Where it is absent, they will create it.

Barrett's account is a typical narrative found in most modern psychiatric services. It is very serviceable for our current state of knowledge of schizophrenia. Of course, things do not always go well with the treatment of schizophrenia. Then the trajectory is different, heading towards chronic schizophrenia. The capacity to see the patient as a full person remains diminished, and she continues to be seen more in terms of illness-causation, and less as a self-determining being. Other patients might lead to other narratives. For instance, the following is not uncommon (this is a different kind of patient, not a psychotic one, to demonstrate the variety of psychiatric narratives):

> A 29-year-old woman was admitted to a mental hospital, depressed and apparently suicidal. She spoke very little to the admitting doctor; she seemed hopeless and put herself completely in his hands. He felt sympathetic to the dejected figure in front of him and diagnosed a suicidal psychotic depression. Within a couple of days she became brighter, but more demanding. She was talkative with other patients. The staff felt heartened by this dramatic response to their care and considered her a depressed neurotic. Quickly she became very helpful to the staff, but then gradually more and more intrusive and controlling in the life of the ward. This helpful patient became more difficult; she controlled her own life, her medication and her movements. She recruited other patients to her schemes. Among the staff, discussions about her pleasing recovery began to fade. They began to wonder how depressed she had really been when she came into the ward. Instead, they now thought that when she had presented herself as depressed and suicidal it had been over-dramatic. Soon she was called manipulative, and eventually hysterical. There were increasing confrontations between her and the staff over the ward rules and customs. From this point, the patient became less and less helpful, and she lost the support of other patients. Staff meetings increasingly expressed frustration with this patient. The doctors were criticised for being too permissive with her. Finally this troublesome patient was regarded as not deserving admission. The doctors labelled her a personality disorder, and discharged her.

In this sequence, over about three and a half weeks the diagnosis was progressively revised, with an increasingly strong negative tone to the relationship with the patient. The diagnosis became a means of expressing an increasing degree of negativity: from suicidal depressive, to neurotic depressive, to manipulative hysteric, and finally a psychopathic personality disorder. There is a narrative to the course of this admission, although it is a different narrative from that of the typical schizophrenic one. In this case, the patient tended to retain from the beginning of the admission a 'moral' status, unlike a schizophrenic; this patient was someone responsible for herself. Her progress was therefore in terms of the moral value given to her as a person – from object of pity, to helpfulness, to demanding manipulation. The staff moved from liking to disliking her, and the diagnosis changed accordingly. This is another trajectory in which meaning is constructed at each stage – especially meaning in the form of a diagnosis. Because of the restless need in psychiatry to construct meaning, these narratives are a part of the psychology of carers, but separate from the professional attempts at a scientific diagnosis and treatment. The psychology of care and the professional work become mixed. In both this case and a patient with schizophrenia, stories are lived out meaningfully by staff and patients.

Caring staff need as much as anything to make sense of their patients and the conditions they suffer from. It is necessary that the sense they make is meaningful and coherent. So often – perhaps always – that sense takes the form of a narrative (Kleinman 1988; Hacking 1999). Whatever the nature of meaning, we need it to make our work satisfying. Psychotic patients so often deny us this satisfaction. Their incoherence and the bewildering meaninglessness of their utterances and behaviour are debilitating. It is not surprising then that staff construct the narrative of an illness in place of the narrative of a person.

Who knows?

The staff's efforts to give meaning are a response to the endemic lack of meaning in schizophrenia. It is like a vacuum, and the mind abhors it, filling it quickly with meaning. The staff's efforts in this respect are not just for the staff; they also impact back on the patient. The psychotic patient comes to rely on staff knowing, *instead of the patient*. For instance, the patient whose admission Conran described (see p. 12) was eventually discharged.

> Two or three years passed. The doctor . . . found himself wondering what had become of the woman. He rather thoughtlessly looked her up in the telephone directory and called a number he supposed possibly hers. The woman answered the telephone

> herself and expressed her delight that he should enquire about her . . . after some exchanges [she] said suddenly – 'What was I doing in that hospital?' The doctor was aghast for the manner of her question seemed to brook no evasion. She repeated the question insistently.
>
> The doctor mumbled something to the effect – 'Well! I rather wondered if you might not be able to tell me that.' 'Me?' she replied, 'Me! How should I know? I expect you to know. You must know. Tell me, what was I doing there all that time' . . . By this time the doctor was wishing he had minded his own business . . . [he] muttered his excuses and said his farewell. (Conran 1985, p. 38)

So, this woman, long after the event, had still shown no recognition of what had been done for her, or even that anything needed to be done. She had still not regained her capacity to comprehend herself and she still insisted that the doctor carry her self-knowing. However, the doctor believed that particular burden of care was over, and he had done his job. While she was in hospital, the doctor had taken over functions of care, understanding and responsibility for her, which should normally have been hers. Now, he merely had an interested concern for her. For the patient that was not enough. She still demanded that the original arrangement with the doctor should persist. From her point of view, the doctor was still responsible, and his voice on the phone became an immediate invitation to resume where she had left off when discharged. The woman allowed no respect for the reality of the doctor's *actual* position, his actual knowledge or his discomfort. He was dramatically forced to see what a thankless task he had.

We can understand something about this lack of appreciation from this vignette. The doctor had an interested concern, but the patient insisted on something else, which he found very difficult to resist. She wanted him to take over responsibility for her self-knowledge. His interest had actually to become her self-care. There is a difference between having a concern for her, as another person, on one hand, and on the other *being* her concern, her self-care, her self-control. In the latter, she is no longer 'another person'. Somehow he is implicated in being some essential part of her; and he is no longer his own person either. He is, as it were, pressed into service as some part of her, and he felt this acutely when she demanded this, even over the phone. Actually *being* some aspect of the patient made it difficult for him to be himself. In her eyes, he was not in fact himself, and therefore not a candidate for her appreciation. She drew him into her own self-interest. And there was no place for his. This is not an ordinary relationship between two people. There was something intensely personal, even intimate, as it involved both of them in some deformation of their identities. As with responsibility, the staff *become* the patient's responsibility, so with knowledge of the patient. Staff are expected to *be* the patient's self-knowledge, and to create it and carry it for him.

Action and understanding

Part of the patient's problem in knowing himself, and separating his self-created delusions and hallucinations from the real world, is that he lost the capacity for effective abstract thought and the use of symbols. This significantly adds to the difficulty in making sense of the experience in psychiatric work. Symbolic thought is downgraded. In Conran's description of his discomfort on the phone (see above), it was clear how much important communication took place outside the symbolic world. The patient with schizophrenia has considerable difficulties with symbols – creating them, using them and understanding them. Instead he uses symbols in a disturbing manner. A symbol normally represents the thing it symbolises; it is not identical to that thing. Schizophrenic people, however, proceed as if the symbol is actually what it symbolises. There is no proper representation, and no proper distinction between the symbol and what is symbolised.

In a famous example, described by Segal (1957), the word 'stool' attracts all the embarrassment and disgust that a piece of faeces would (see also 'Projective identification and symbolic relations' in Essay 2, p. 67). An everyday example is that some Christians believe that at Mass the bread actually becomes the flesh of Christ. There is no metaphor. Without symbolisation, the capacity to think, reflect, generate meaning, and communicate understanding is significantly more difficult (Hinshelwood 2001). Symbols no longer communicate, they become actions upon another person. More than that, in an acute psychotic state, a patient's actions invariably recruit someone else to be a part of the patient's own person – his self-control for instance, or his self-knowledge. Some aspect of the patient's personality, or some part of his self, is relocated outside him, and inside someone else. That directing outwards gives the sense of an action having as its purpose this outward evacuation.

The term 'acting-out' is a way of indicating a kind of mental action that eliminates some mental part or function. In this way, we tend to suffer the insanity of our patients, as the doctor in Conran's paper did when he phoned his patient long after discharge. He was confounded and discomforted, and had to know how disconcerting it was to be filled with the incomprehension once more.

Therefore, it is very difficult to communicate normally in a world of schizophrenia. We must handle non-symbolised utterances and expressions. If non-verbal communications cannot be converted into some form of symbolic communication, we must operate and communicate in non-verbal actions. Such communication requires sensitive intuition, practice, and confidence, because it intrudes into our being, and maybe even abuses us. It requires a good deal of self-composure and self-knowledge on the part of the staff (see Barnes *et al.* 1998 for a discussion of the 'use of self' in psychiatric care). After all, when we receive a schizophrenic communication, we know it through playing some part in the patient's own internal state – like becoming the one who knows, the one who has the patient's self-knowledge; or the one who is responsible, the one who has the patient's self-control and self-care.

Some of these skills can be learned, mostly by example and while on the job, but it depends so much on inherent personal aptitude and intuition. It is the most difficult of all areas of psychiatry to learn – and in which to be trained. It entails, largely, learning through symbolic means about non-symbolic schizophrenic action. The feelings, the problems of identity, and the accurate recognition of other minds are known to us through their impact rather than as articulate statements. The difficulties of proceeding to think in this modality, and then to convey one's thoughts in actions, always compromise the care of schizophrenic people (Hinshelwood 1987c). Thinking and understanding in an action mode is the opportunity available to the psychiatric carer, and that opportunity can seem immensely obscure. Action contrasts with communication, yet in schizophrenia action is the mode of communication.

At the same time, communication can be an action. To communicate an understanding of someone is a kind of act upon that person. In fact, in either of these modes – actions or words – the very fact of understanding someone has an effect on the situation that is understood. Once understood, that person is no longer a misunderstood or incomprehensible mind. It is now a mind in a different state. This cannot be said about mechanical troubles with a car – a car stays immobile, however well you understand its problem. A state of mind has a very special correlation with understanding and being understood. To share a problem with someone who evidently understands is a lever for change. It is a verbal 'medication'. When it comes to feeling understood, staff are no different from patients – and that is important in a psychology of care.

If we deal with a mind as a mechanical entity, it short-circuits personal experience. It is possible to modify mental states with chemical substances, not least alcohol, of course. Pharmaceutical products have alleviated enormous amounts of psychic pain. It is a specifically psychiatric form of understanding that arises from the examination and diagnosis of the mental state. Personal experience is converted into general categories.

So, there is a wide landscape of various forms of understanding and making sense of the incomprehensible schizophrenia:

- first is the natural attempt to listen into the experience that most of us assume is being expressed by another person. That natural empathy is confounded in schizophrenia;
- then there is the professional understanding that relies on categories (diagnoses), bypasses normal empathy, and in the process may depersonalise the patient;
- finally, there is the odd non-symbolic method of communicating through action on another person's mind. Although this kind of emotional impact occurs in all human communication, there is no parallel verbal commentary. In fact, words themselves lose their symbolic nature, and become actions.

This number of modes of communication and understanding makes the work complex, and leaves us confused sometimes as to when a mode is relevant and how to use it.

Identity and meaning are the problems psychotics bring. We can turn now to the 'problems' that are brought into the work by caring staff and their impact on patients.

The professional super-ego

Unfortunately, despite the best motivations, the generally oppressive nature of institutionalised care has rendered countless people over many generations into semi-vegetables. Nobody condones that, and it has been a major factor in the rethinking of psychiatry over the past half-century. It prompted the closure of mental hospitals themselves (see Hinshelwood 2001). However, part of the oppressive atmosphere comes from the demands that staff invariably put upon themselves when they enter a psychiatric career.

The need to care

Donati (1989) described a ward meeting instituted on a long-stay male ward for the purpose of stimulating more normal social contact, relations and activity among the patients. The charge nurse was chairperson of the meeting. He was desperate to promote participation by the patients, but as soon as a patient brought up something serious, either it was a matter for the doctor or it had no solution. The anxious staff member was a deadening hand, anxious that his patients should interact, and at the same time too anxious to let it happen. Human contact, though consciously sought, was suffocated out of existence. The process of stereotyping patients as helpless, inert and inactive had a momentum of its own that made gainsaying it futile. Something went on in the charge nurse to ensure that he obstructed the very thing he thought he wanted to achieve. He thwarted his own efforts to bring his patients, and his ward, to life.

So there was something conflicted in the motivation of the charge nurse. He wanted to help his patients to a more normal manner of living, but in addition he needed to keep the stereotyped roles in place. Moreover, the charge nurse's two motivations were characterised by one being conscious (to enliven his patients socially) while the other (keeping up the stereotypes) appeared to be unconscious. It is the unconscious motivation involved in care that I shall concentrate on now.

Unconscious motivations

There is more to the unconscious motivation than keeping up stereotypes. We need to look further into the feelings about the work. Each kind of work will bring up different discomforts. Working in a coalmine makes miners feel insecure due to accidents, and the diseases they can eventually get. Working in a factory that makes nuclear weapons will arouse other feelings – about the enormity of the destructive power they bring into being. Educationalists will have worries in accordance with their view of children – whether they are very vulnerable and need protection, or whether they are very destructive beings and need to be controlled and restricted to adult types of behaviour.

Menzies (1959), in a classic paper, described a specific anxiety in healthcare, one that comes from witnessing the suffering, mutilation and death of patients. Running alongside this conscious wish to nurse and care is a primitive level of phantasy[3] about the suffering that the nurse tries to alleviate:

> the objective situation confronting the nurse bears a striking resemblance to the phantasy situations that exist in every individual in the deepest and most primitive levels of the mind. (Menzies 1959, p. 440)

At the unconscious level there are phantastical views, experiences and motives regarding ill and damaged human beings. These conceptions may be a long way from the reality, just as they are a long way from being conscious. At that unconscious level of phantasy, illness is conceived in the most lurid forms of pain, danger and damage. Sometimes patients are, in fact, desperately ill or injured, and come close to these unconscious phantasies. The combination of patients and those phantasies arouses high levels of fear, anxiety and guilt; and in turn a powerful responsibility for the sick.

These deep-seated phantasies and feelings are connected with deep concerns about doing violence, and damage. Being deep they are rarely fully confronted, though they may be titillated through film, theatre and novels, or news-reporting on television. These violent phantasies are not just the basis for enjoying horror movies, or murder stories; they also cause our tendency to feel concern for each other. Care and concern are a reaction to secret evil we have in our hearts. (These feelings constitute what Melanie Klein called the depressive position (Klein 1935, 1940).) They are a motivating force, especially to care, as a means for atonement for the violence. However, such complex feelings and motives are rarely consciously known.

Mostly, these feelings of violence and reaction are at a distance from our experience of life. Nurses, however, are confronted directly with people whose pain, fear and damage are intensely present in the room, and who implore their nurses for care and relief. Because their unconscious phantasies are enlivened by this close contact, carers'

3 'Phantasy' is a technical term to denote an unconscious level of operation; 'fantasy' means day-dreaming etc. (see Isaacs 1948).

relations at work become highly stressed. Carers feel unnatural and overwhelming responsibility.

When these unconscious phantasies of dreadful things happening to others are charged up, they call out equally powerful demands on ourselves. We charge ourselves in equal measure to care and repair. One of the characteristics of this unconscious level is that the phantasies tend to have the quality called 'omnipotence'. For instance:

> An analysand in psychoanalysis had a recurrent dream about rats. On one occasion he looked out, in his dream, from his back window and saw the yard and his garden covered in rats. Their numbers were so vast and the extent of them so far that he felt completely overwhelmed by their noxious contamination and relentless gnawing violence.

The overwhelming quality was so powerful that he had absolutely no sense that he could do anything about this invasion. He felt impotent in the face of the overwhelming malevolence. The problem is that with these nightmare phantasies, there is a belief that any concern and reconstructive efforts must be, in like measure, omnipotent, overwhelming, and invincible.

When phantasies and wishes like this are remote from our conscious appreciation they can easily have an 'omnipotent' overwhelming quality. Actual nightmares allow us to look around when we wake to make sure that the dream is not real, but the unconscious phantasies (of destruction) and wishes (to repair) are like dreams from which we do not wake. They determine a level of feeling, anxiety and motivation which drive us, but we do not wake up to how real they might be – or how unrealistic. In fact, patients do sometimes die; they may be in pain that can only be partially relieved. Their fears may not be possible to reassure. Sometimes accidents do seriously mutilate them; mutilating operations may have to be performed. These are realities, and in some branches of healthcare they are everyday realities, that cannot be avoided. Care is not omnipotent and cannot heal everything. Without realistic assessment, there is a risk of becoming disheartened, burnt-out or depressed. The source of that ill-ease is the level of unreality that operates within us, and demands of us achievements we cannot produce.

Specific anxieties in mental health correspond to these anxieties involving care of the physically and bodily sick. Anxieties in psychiatry are rather different from general medicine. The anxiety in mental healthcare is more to do with a damaged and destroyed mind and person, rather than destroyed bodies. There is a fear of the mad as potentially violent, and in addition a fear of infection by the madness of the patients, including their meaninglessness. And above all we need to care for such people. However, as in general medicine, transferred from phantasies onto patients, the demands on ourselves to care and cure are not necessarily realistic.

There is therefore a significant component of the work experience and of the job satisfaction that comes from this 'primitive' level rather than from a sophisticated view of the problems to be solved. (This primitive level of unrealistic phantasy is often called 'infantile', on the supposition that a baby, as yet unable to grasp reality fully, is occupied, and a prey to, its own phantasies of what is happening to it and to its world. We, in our primitive levels, are similarly a prey to unconscious phantasies that are not challenged by reality.) Being unconscious, this level of motivation is difficult to address in a realistic and sophisticated way, and we become trapped with demands of ourselves that are quite unrealistic. There are then important consequences to our omnipotent and unrealistic expectations of what we can do, and repair. In psychoanalytic terms the super-ego issues a powerful imperative, pressing us on to do better and better. In the context of these disastrous phantasies, the super-ego can be very severe, a taskmaster impossible to appease, which creates a continual bad conscience about one's performance and achievement at work.

Hatred and guilt

If we have impossible omnipotent demands of ourselves, in our hearts, then it will not be long before we have to cope with the inability to meet those demands. That is, we have to experience failure. In the work context, guilt is closely connected with failure. We are paid to succeed, and we have our own deep and primitive psychological motivations to succeed. When we do not, and we fail, that impacts on our view of ourselves. We have to suffer a guilt about our financial rewards when we fail; moreover, we have to appease our super-ego, which embodies our omnipotent, even magical, demands to restore severely damaged patients to health and happiness.

Unlike many other branches of medicine, psychiatric failures very often live long lives. Even the successes often live very impoverished lives. Success in psychiatry needs to be carefully scaled. It is a relative measure. So many patients do not get better in the ordinary sense. We need to assess degrees of improvement – often very small degrees – rather than cures. Even those small degrees of improvement can be significant achievements for some patients, and should therefore count as significant successes for staff. Our job is to grasp a complex reality – the reality of the patient's condition, the reality of our stress, and the reality of relative improvements. Against this is ranged the reality of our need to care to perfectionist standards, and of our persecuting guilt when we do not.

We as staff are very vulnerable to our internal standards, demands and criticisms, and guilt is very much present on the sidelines. Guilt can come easily and crushingly if we do not take psychological steps to protect ourselves. Looking again at the example of the 29-year old suicidal woman who was discharged as a psychopath (see p. 17), that narrative is one in which staff modified the diagnosis progressively as a result of primitive forces that led them from sympathy, via failure and irritation, to condemnation. The condemning criticism with which staff might beat themselves for not succeeding comes to be turned into condemnation of the patient.

Staff (like anyone) commonly turn their hopes into anger against the people who make them feel failures. Staff, vulnerable to their own feelings, modify them impulsively in this and other ways. Sadly, they end up hating the people they are most motivated to help and cure. It is very hard for carers to feel hatred for their charges. Love is implicit in the general notion of care – not hate. So, the common method of evading a sense of failure (anger and hate) results in an emotional state that carers feel is the antithesis of what they *should* be feeling. Thus, when they get angry, they then have another burst of criticism from their professional super-egos. In turn, they feel more desperate, and focus their need on their patients to make them feel successes. Such an increasing need of their patients coexists with feeling an angry rejection of them. This is a very difficult intensifying ambivalence to have to tolerate. Yet such is the oddity of our patients, and the motivational needs of the staff, that painfully mixed feelings like this are not uncommon.

We can recall Winnicott's startling paper 'Hate in the countertransference' (Winnicott 1949). He asserts that hate is a normal part of the treatment of patients, especially seriously ill patients; but he goes further and states that 'The mother, however, hates her infant from the word go' (p. 73). This is a very challenging statement. And yet mothers do have a hard time being a mother, and that is probably true of absolutely every mother. They can succumb occasionally to hatred of their baby, who causes mother to suffer. Psychiatric staff are like mothers in this respect, as Winnicott says. They need their patients, like mothers need their children, to give them reassurance, and to act as a buffer against the activity of the self-demands from their professional super-ego. Instead, patients give them a hard time.

Emotional vulnerability

I have drawn attention to the phenomenon of a professional super-ego as a source of negative feelings towards patients. However, it is not the only source, and perhaps not the strongest and most prevalent source. Just as important is the fact that our patients may themselves actually be hateful. They may have a lot of anger to discharge. Increasingly as our wards concentrate more disturbed people in a confined space, there is increasing risk, and fear. The most obvious fear is about physical violence that staff will have to face with their patients. Working with very disturbed or psychotic people does usually mean working with a level of physical violence that is potentially a real threat, and therefore frightening. However, physical violence is not the only fear, and perhaps not the worst one. Another fear is of madness itself and the contagion. We should not forget that there is a kind of emotional contagion, as we saw earlier in this essay, in which parts of mad people can actually infiltrate into the identity of carers and others.

One aspect of the fear of infection is a fear of our own madness, so that when our psychiatric institutions assert that patients are mad and staff are sane, it is relieving and reassuring. These attitudes make the staff feel more comfortable about themselves. Staff can be quite disturbed in their emotions – not least by the stress of the work. A psychotic patient does cause stress with the burdens of responsibility and of knowing. He causes a painful confusion of personal identity – a confusion about who he is, and who the carer is. So, the work can be seriously disturbing, even maddening. At the same time the expectation is that staff must function as examples of sanity, just as they should be eternally loving in the face of the worst. They will demand of themselves that they live up to that standard prescribed by cultural expectations – sane staff and mad patients.

Working in psychiatry and treating psychotic patients inevitably causes a turmoil of feeling inside you. Yet it is one of the biggest fears that such turmoil and madness is your own madness. One staff reaction is to pretend we are not disturbed or upset by the work. Often there is an expectation that psychiatric staff remain undisturbed and unmoved, and must maintain the countenance of someone who is perfectly undisturbed, all of the time. In fact, of course, they are troubled by their patients, yet it cannot be properly talked about among the team, because of their professional superego's expectation of calmness and sanity. Staff may then fail to support each other. So members of staff are very lonely with their troubled feelings.

If the staff could think about the way they are upset by their patients, they could learn a lot about the patients. The specific fears and anger the staff member feels point to specific fears and aggression in the patient – for instance, a burden of responsibility may derive from the patient's loss of self-control, which may need to be directly addressed. However, because staff cannot admit to these feelings – either to themselves or to each other – something of what they could know gets lost.

Other things happen, too. Staff develop many ways in which they can deal with their experience of patients. Often the first thing is to project those feelings back into their patients, usually with a very powerful reaction from the patient. For instance, if a patient makes a member of staff feel guilty, then the staff member may immediately put the responsibility back onto the patient – to make him feel guilty. The patient may then react very strongly, by complaining, or with violence, or an exacerbation of his symptoms – perhaps until the staff deal with the situation with sedative drugs.

Aggression and negativity

Patients feel aggressive and become violent for many reasons. The most important cause is actually the least obvious, and therefore the most neglected. This is the patients' own underlying feeling of fear and vulnerability. It is neglected because people who are violent do not appear fearful or vulnerable. In fact they may often seem the most courageous, indeed foolishly so, but the violence and the bravery are ways of denying the fear and vulnerability. In our hostels, hospitals, and communities, our clients and patients are in fact vulnerable. They feel no real power or control, and realistically they are helpless because they have so often split off and projected their own initiative and agency. A common cycle occurs in which someone who is difficult is marked down by the staff for transfer. This provokes the client's insecurity, as the impending transfer stimulates his feeling of helplessness and vulnerability. That results in more aggression as a denial of his vulnerability, and then staff have more urgency about transferring him.

Violence is in fact dangerous whatever its source. Such an obvious fact is obvious *to the patient* as well – in some corner of his mind. So, very often in psychiatry patients feel in need of a controlling agency from outside themselves, and the patient may be as reassured as the staff by effective control of himself – even by the police (see below). The patient is on a search for someone to *be* his self-control. The patient may therefore feel less secure if he is not adequately controlled, an insecurity which will in turn fuel his dangerousness.

Besides the realistic vulnerability of our clients, and the power that we have over their lives in our institutions, there is another kind of vulnerability that is more important to the client and again is often not easily seen by the staff. This is their emotional vulnerability. It is a very common reason for verbal and emotional aggression. Very many of the people we care for suffer an intense and uncontrolled emotional life. They can be said to be vulnerable *to their own feelings*. Once psychiatric patients are sufficiently able to experience their feelings, they feel them to be intolerable – jealousy, exclusion, rivalry, frustration, etc. They may then be explosively emotional, dangerous, or deluded and hallucinated. Very often the illness that results in their admission to our institutions is something to do with the means of coping with such intolerable feelings.

So, there is a vulnerability that has to do with their psychological state, and not just their physical, bodily safety. Anything that threatens to arouse a feeling state which they believe is unbearable is therefore very powerful, and they feel vulnerable to it. The following is an example.

> A man in hospital was very frightened of going to bed at night. He did have bad dreams but he claimed there was something else, much worse, which he could not specify. He was in effect phobic about his bed, and he would delay going to bed at night well after the time required. He was always very aggressive verbally. This got him into a lot of trouble, and staff and clients were annoyed with the disturbances every night. Eventually, in the course of psychotherapy, it emerged that he had powerful homosexual feelings. These feelings threatened to be aroused by sleeping with a male room-mate. In effect the close sleeping

> arrangement threatened this man because of powerful sexual wishes, which he could not own (at first). When he negotiated a single room, for three weeks, he was much calmer. Subsequently, when he returned to the room with the other man, he could manage his emotional state better.

The point is that this man's feelings could overwhelm him, and he was therefore vulnerable to them. In his case it was a phobic reaction to the bed in his bedroom, and led to meaningless fears of aggression.

Emotional vulnerability is quite a common experience for everyone. Merely being in love, for instance, may overwhelm us with feelings of need – needing the loved one. Then the following disastrous situation can arise: as the need to see or be with the loved one increases, so the internal state intensifies. Tension and perhaps jealousy or exclusion come more and more to the fore. The lover becomes in that moment a threat, the one who arouses the emotional pain, dependence and vulnerability. As a result the lover can become feared, someone who threatens, and ultimately someone who may have to be treated as an enemy! The love has, through fear and vulnerability, turned to aggression. For many people who come to us for help, their past, particularly as a child, has been with carers whom the child has loved but who have aroused intolerable deprivation, so that all love and care turns quickly to hate and revenge.

We, as staff, are also emotionally vulnerable, and we too can react with annoyance. Overt violence is obvious, and we must act to protect ourselves. However, we do not react just with self-protection, but usually with fear and a retaliatory aggression as well. It happens in ordinary life. Imagine two people driving cars that hit each other. They immediately jump out and attack each other verbally. One driver immediately shouts and abuses the other in order to deal with his own feelings of hurt or guilt or fear. And the other, out of fear and guilt and anger, retaliates in the same way, making the first one more afraid and angry. In this way they build up a crescendo of anxiety and aggression, each trying to make the other person feel bad and frightened. This cycle escalates because, when the frightened person makes his attacks, he then feels afraid of retaliation. In turn, the person who has been attacked wants to attack back and may actually do so. So the cycle that goes on inside the person may be accelerated by what happens inside the other person. A spiralling situation can lead to greater and greater forms of violence and aggression. Often we condemn the patient for making us aggressive: in other words, we tend to meet aggression with an aggressive reaction in ourselves.

This is not to say that we should not have such reactions to our clients. They are quite natural. In fact, anyone who claimed she did not feel aggression and hatred would most likely be denying her actual fear and aggression. Nevertheless, it is very tempting to deny that we are angry with the people we care for.

Disguised aggression

Besides overt threats, there are also many subtle forms of aggressiveness. The innumerable methods of quiet defiance, undermining, and 'passive aggression' may be much harder to spot. At times we may have to accept that even not getting better may be the expression of some negative emotional state (the 'negative therapeutic reaction'). These are particularly difficult strategies for staff, because they often leave us feeling frustrated and annoyed without being able to define clearly how the client has annoyed us. An example is the well-known phenomenon of splitting the staff. A client will relate to one staff member in a very positive way, making her or him feel good, while another is compared unfavourably with the first staff member (Main 1957). Staff end up quarrelling with each other. Alternatively, the 'approved of' staff member loses favour and is then compared, badly, with a third staff member. The first staff member feels a very sudden loss, and is vulnerable to failure, guilt, etc., which may evoke an angry reaction. These are subtle ways of attacking the confidence and the motivation of staff, and thus of expressing subtle aggression.

Aggression can be communicated through non-verbal kinds of communication. As we saw above, psychotic patients in particular communicate their feelings directly to other people. Our patients can try to communicate to us how frightened they are by trying to make us feel frightened. A patient wants to make the other person know how she feels by making the other person feel it. This is a very important and very hidden form of psychological interaction, and our patients very often use us to communicate with in this kind of way. It is often very difficult to understand that the patient is making a communication about her feelings. Part of the difficulty is that this process feels very aggressive and we don't like patients intruding on us like this. We may say 'they are very manipulative', as with the suicidal woman reported above. They do manipulate our minds: they manipulate in order to communicate. If a patient continually tries to communicate by making you feel frightened, it feels very much as if you are under an attack from which you feel fear. So in a way we fail to understand what the patient is doing – communicating – and react by becoming defensive, as if she were attacking. Then the patient feels you have not understood her communication and believes that you don't know how she feels, so she may try to make her communication stronger, and hence you feel even more unpleasantly interfered with in your feelings. So, you proceed in a state of non-communication which becomes more aggressive as the patient tries more forcefully to make you feel what she feels. It becomes increasingly difficult to decide whether a patient is trying to communicate or trying to hurt. Yet it is vital to try to do so. It is vital to the patient that you help her to identify her communicating as distinct from her aggression.

I have concentrated more on patients' negative feelings and on these negative situations, but patients can, of course, feel the full range of positive emotions too, and these may also cause difficulties for a carer, when exaggerated and sexual, for instance. Patients can genuinely respect and feel grateful to staff in large measure and often have caring impulses for them too. These positive feelings may often be very hidden. So, we reach the sad situation when clients hide their positive feelings behind hateful ones, and staff struggle to hide their aggression behind a bland but unconvincing positive demeanour.

Contagion and boundaries

Often caught in the trap of feeling increasingly angry and frightened, while strictly prohibited from revealing their frustrated anger, staff exist in a very uncomfortable emotional predicament – a lonely ambivalence. Because it is inexpressible, staff feel very isolated, and begin to suspect their own sanity. Then the boundary between being a patient and being staff erodes. Normally that boundary is reassuringly high and unbreachable, because of the stereotypes. But if that stereotyping becomes eroded, staff can begin to feel a loss of the identity of a healthy member of staff. This occurred poignantly in the following example.

> A 35-year-old psychologist was admitted to a psychotherapeutic community as an emergency after she had been attacked with a

knife by one of her patients. She was not injured but had been held a prisoner in her room by the patient for one hour.

The psychologist was a difficult patient. She became extremely angry with several other patients in a small group that she was part of. On one occasion, she entered the bedroom of another patient and took a screw out of his bed so that it collapsed. In the ward, she saw a psychotherapist individually once a week; he found it very difficult to keep his attention on what she said and felt that his mind became confused. At times he felt uncomfortable because he noticed strong feelings towards her.

In her history, she had been sent away to a boarding school when she was 12 years old. She was very distressed at school. Previously she had been the youngest and favourite child in the family. She believed that when she was newborn her mother had been very worried and preoccupied by the illness of an older sister. It was noticed while she was in the ward that when she was distressed she often developed bodily symptoms – notably pain which she said came from her womb.

In treating his patient, the psychotherapist became very uncomfortable and found that his thinking became confused. Part of the psychotherapist's discomfort was, it seemed, because he was treating a psychiatric professional who had become a patient. This raised anxieties in him. He described feeling lost, feeling strangely attracted to her, and also confused by what she was trying to say. He described it as a 'crazy-paving' case, because nothing fitted together properly.

The psychologist who became a patient expressed her feelings about breaking down by making her psychotherapist's mind confused, and broken up like crazy-paving. In addition, she made another patient's bed break. The therapist could eventually understand that the patient's most important fears were about her own mind and how it had failed her and broken down. She made an intrusion into the therapist's mind. She caused him to feel that he was coming apart in crazy pieces and breaking down.

This patient had been subjected to an intense fear by the attack from one of her own patients. Triggered by that experience, she became paranoid and violent. The fear resulted in such a disturbance in her that she became difficult, broke down, and eventually in the hospital she too attacked people. She verbally attacked people in the patients' group, who seemed to make her angry; she was physically aggressive when she went into someone's bedroom and broke his bed. These are two kinds of aggression – verbal aggression and physical violence.

However, a third form of aggression occurred in this case. She intruded into the therapist's mind just as into the other patient's bedroom. Thus, the psychotherapist's mind was disturbed by the patient. That is an interesting process. The clear stereotypes were dissolving: the patient was herself a psychologist who worked with patients, and her mind broke down. What she did with her psychotherapist was, in a way, to make his mind break down. We see here the process by which a patient can get into the therapist's mind and spread confusion there. The psychotherapist had been infected, as it were, by the patient's contagion. This felt very intrusive for the psychotherapist, a projective process into his mind, causing discomfort. The carer had to suffer, and was vulnerable, because the stereotype figures of patient and staff had became blurred due to the patient's actual profession.

The effect of the staff vulnerability is also interesting. Through the patient's intrusion into the therapist she made a kind of communication. When she went into someone's bedroom and made their bed collapse, it was similar to when someone (a man with a knife) came into her room and made her collapse. So, it is a communication, misdirected perhaps, to the person whose room she went into. She had felt intruded upon in a very physical way: so much so that it became bodily, and she felt pain inside her body, in her womb. This patient was so disturbed that her ability to use ordinary symbolic communication failed her. She had to substitute physical and bodily acts – the pain in her womb, the intrusion into someone's bedroom, sowing confusion in her psychotherapist's mind. They all probably represent something like rape, but could not be expressed symbolically as in the words I just used. She had to communicate the experience by doing it to someone else. This method depends on disturbing another person, while it is so difficult for staff to admit that they are disturbed. So, staff cannot always use the knowledge that their own feelings could bring them.

There is a sadness as individual staff go about their work labouring with the same feelings, but isolated in non-communication with each other, because they are not expected to feel disturbed. They are isolated from the patients' communication, because they lack the support of colleagues that might help them to find words for these intruded feelings. Unfortunately, these features of the psychology of the staff are not studied enough. As a result, staff suffer in isolation. This is regrettable, because the intrusions could also be informative. Effectiveness in the job diminishes, and with it, inevitably, job satisfaction.

Unconscious job satisfaction

I want to concentrate on one of the consequences in particular. When we do our job and achieve results, it is a source of satisfaction. I shall leave aside the financial rewards, and the social rewards of having friends in the team. Also, I am not dwelling on career-building, which is important for many people. For everyone, a satisfaction comes from the performance and results of the work. However, like everything else in life, the results are only likely to be good to a certain degree. Nothing is ever perfect. 'Good-enough' is what we must live with, but this is a sophisticated expectation – to do a job well enough. It is a different matter when we come to the unconscious level. There, unreality dominates and, as we have seen, exaggerated results are expected. The job must be perfectly done (omnipotently); in our case the clients must be restored to perfect sanity, but we find only imperfection. In mental healthcare there is inevitably a lot of feelings of failure floating around, and our services are particularly prone to being undermined by such feelings. All workers depend in part on their own standards, and in part on appreciation by those they serve.

Job satisfaction is a fragile thing in mental health, and can be in short supply. The reasons are as follows.

- Staff get less direct appreciative response from their patients than other carers do.
- They are infected with especially difficult feelings of incomprehension and meaninglessness, and of responsibility for the patient's own responsibility, as we have seen.
- The expectations staff have of themselves are often exaggerated by 'primitive' omnipotent phantasies that are unrealisable, and therefore undermine confidence in a way that is not properly recognised.
- Only with a proper and therefore vulnerable contact with the patient can any sense of realistic achievement be enjoyed.

In addition, many of the things that undermine job satisfaction cannot be spoken to each other, and often staff cannot express them to themselves properly either. They remain isolated areas within the carers' minds, and they can fester there.

The neglected psychology

General attitudes encourage staff to believe that their own feelings and experiences should not be acknowledged. Why is this a neglected area of psychology? There are probably several factors in the answer.

1 *Emotional distance*: The fear of madness demands that staff keep as distant as possible in order to avoid provoking violence, and in order to avoid contamination (and unconsciously the peculiar concrete projections of schizophrenic patients). Characteristically, staff avoid emotional contact and engagement (as with the charge nurse described by Donati (1989) – see p. 23), and this is a widespread implicit attitude and style of doing the work (see Essay 3 for a discussion of psychiatric cultures).
2 *A blind eye*: Staff psychology is simply overlooked, because we do not expect it. The radical distinction between patients and staff suggests that staff are invulnerable, hence staff stress should be insignificant and can be ignored. Hence, we do not see staff stress until it reaches a high level of urgency. The stereotyped view of staff and patients is persuasive because it offers some sort of comfort for staff, and may be needed by patients. The potential stress is so fearsome to contemplate that it is dealt with by simply turning a blind eye. In planning services, as in providing them, we blank out staff stress.
3 *Rationality*: Based on the assumption of staff invulnerability, all problems will be rational ones. The irrational is dealt with as if it does not exist. Rational solutions are all that is necessary. Irrational problems belong to patients and not to the staff in our institutions. Rational solutions take the form of structural rearrangements, implementing procedures, or quantifying of resources and their reallocation. The emotional level is rarely treated as a problem, and could only attract irrelevant rational solutions in a rationalist culture.
4 *Management style*: Outside healthcare, the dominant mode of management is 'scientific management', which equally applauds reason (Taylor 1911; see also de Vries 1991; Stapley 1996). So, when imported into the mental health services, this has married

with the need from within to stick to reason (this is considered in detail under 'Scientific management' in Essay 3, p. 145). Collusion at this level between managers and psychiatric clinicians impoverishes or abolishes all categories with which to think about staff stress.

This list of factors is certainly incomplete, but it is a first step towards thinking about the neglected psychology. First staff must be aware of it; then, we must be aware that staff psychology is an emotional psychology, not a rational one, and that staff can be vulnerable, just as patients are.

However, exhortation to be aware is not a great success against the powerful forces that turn us away, that demand a blind eye, that deny staff stress, and that put up the seductive barrier of stereotypes. Acceptance of staff stress must involve an abandonment of the dichotomous view that patients are disturbed and staff are not. Unconscious forces protect that view. The polarisation of staff as healthy and wise, and patients as ignorant and unhealthy, is an unconscious product of the stress inherent in the work. Given that the work is with people who have been admitted because they have found stress intolerable, it is not surprising that a similar fear of stress infects the whole institution. It is true that the task *feels* large – grotesquely, impossibly and omnipotently large. It is all too understandable to back away feeling hopeless – as do our patients. Moreover, it is equally understandable to dash overconfidently for simplistic answers. Maybe the simple plan of closing all the old mental hospitals and relying on medications was one of those simplistic answers. Instead, sober reassessment has become necessary. We need a long hard look at what is practicable, and that must include an assessment of unconscious determinants of stress. We might want to consider, given the omnipotence of unconscious thinking, that the reality of the task may not be as insurmountable or daunting as it unconsciously feels.

Reflective practice

I have discussed the impact of psychosis in which meaning and identity are corrupted or dismantled, which gives rise to the special need to support responsibility and understanding. Then what should be done? In a general way, we can say that staff need support, even though the ethos of the psychiatric service blinds staff to that need.

If staff are adequately supported they will be less likely to promote stereotyped roles, distort identity, suffer from confusion and meaninglessness, or protect themselves behind distancing attitudes to the work and to their patients. But what kind of support would this be?

We must be careful. If we look at the problem we have uncovered, it is not exactly that the staff need reassurance – after all, unconscious dynamics fill up their minds with the sense of being powerful helpers ('healthy, knowledgeable, kind, powerful and active' said Tom Main (1975) – see 'Institutionalisation', p. 13). That is already all the reassurance that could be given. It is no good saying to the staff simply, 'Oh, you are doing a good job'. That is not what is needed. The sense of failure has been dispelled already by concentrating on how very different we are from patients. Despite staff being somewhat similar to the patients – distressed, beset by meaninglessness, overburdened with unrealistic responsibility, and operating with unconscious and primitive ways of relating, thinking and symbolising – our defensive attitudes shield us through giving the *feeling* that we are different. We jointly construct our own sense of being helpers, invulnerable and omnipotent, while the patients carry the feelings of being mad and helpless. So, support cannot consist of telling the staff what they have already constructed. To reassure staff that they are natural and wonderful helpers simply feeds into the protective and unrealistic system of stereotypes and feelings.

The opposite, though, is severely problematic too. If, instead of being reassured, staff are criticised, it will play on their feeling of failure. That, in turn, will reinforce the means of coping, i.e. the clinging to the stereotype of health and success will intensify. We are back to square one.

However, it is obvious that the staff's unconscious and omnipotent ambition to cure their patients must fail, because the impulses to repair are unrealistic. Moreover, if staff insist on curing themselves by attributing failure to patients, the solution creates an obvious new problem. That defensive need to stereotype patients as hopeless failures contradicts the wish to turn damaged people back into perfect health. The staff's belief that patients are hopeless inherently contradicts the ambition. Such a contradiction is typical of a neurotic solution, and the result is that the hidden unconscious quality of the solution leads to an equally hidden sense of something being not quite right with the way things are.

So, what kind of support is needed? The contradictory and unconscious knot needs to be cut through.

What to do

The staff's solution to their stress, we have noted, is to resort to a 'primitive' level of mental functioning – stereotyping patients. The characteristic of that protective defence is that these phantasy roles are not adequately connected and checked against reality. We are, by virtue of the unconscious pressures, only partially tied down to the real world. Armed with this argument, we can pinpoint what an effective help would be. Effective help for staff would be to deal with this unreality, to help strengthen a *realistic* appraisal of the situation. A realistic appraisal would require assessment of the actual degree of hope, the actual degree of helplessness of the patients, the realistic change that can be achieved, and in addition, promoting an awareness of some of the realistic vulnerability of the staff.

If we understand the particular kind of unconscious protective solution, then the support that is needed must focus there. Staff need help in disentangling what is real, what is phantasy and what has been created by phantasy. The protective psychodynamics reinforce the illusory stereotypes, so that they become actual reality, and the patients actually become the shuffling, helpless cases that once populated the large mental hospitals. In practice, this means that staff need help in deciding what is a realistic achievement, given the current understanding of mental disorder. They need help in putting that beside their insistent hope to achieve a lot more than what is realistic. In other words, their own unrealistic expectations of themselves need to be set alongside the realities of what can be done successfully. This may be difficult for the staff to recognise. It means that for many patients, hopes can only be limited. However, in the long term, to get hold of the reality of the work has a stabilising effect. Hopes based on unrealistic and unconscious expectations are ultimately self-defeating. In fact, recognising realistic aims and achievements can be a satisfaction in itself.

Effective support in mental health is neither reassurance nor criticism. Effective support is help to recognise reality – to distinguish reality from unrealistic hopes that staff have of themselves, and then of their patients. Helping to support the helpers is helping to understand reality. This reality must be in terms of what we can actually hope for each individual patient – despite the staff aspiring always to unrealistic goals.

To strengthen respect for reality, one kind of intervention is a consultancy. Consultancy is an act merely of understanding these things. It is a process of study, of thinking and understanding. The process may be long, but the ultimate aim is to reveal what is not acknowledged. It comes a step before planning and managing. Understanding is not, therefore, 'doing'. However, understanding is in its effects a powerful act, even before any physical act or decision has been taken.

We commonly accept that 'a trouble shared is a trouble halved'. Understanding, in this sense, is not like finding out what is wrong with the car, and then going to get a new part. When it comes to the mind and the relations it makes with others, understanding has a whole extra dimension. The very fact of understanding someone has an effect on the situation that is understood. Once understood, that person's mind is no longer a misunderstood or incomprehensible mind. It is now a mind in a different state. This cannot be said about understanding the mechanical troubles with a car – a car stays immobile, however well you understand its problem.

To deal with a mind as if it is a mechanical entity is to deny half of its being. Chemical modification of its function is effective in certain ways, but not in those that enhance its human and mental qualities. Drugs may release a mind to be more of a mind, but they do not directly affect its being a mind. To operate directly on a mind involves relating to it with understanding, communicating with meaning, liking and approving or the opposite, to and fro.

Changing states of mind is intimately connected to understanding and being understood. To share a problem with someone who evidently understands is a lever for change. It is a verbal 'medication'. When it comes to feeling understood, staff are no different from patients. This is just as true of the psychology of care; in fact more so, since understanding psychotic patients is so difficult.

If the first item on a 'to-do' list is to recognise the importance of staff psychology, the second item on the list is to give opportunity for a reflective 'space' to address that psychology. Meaning and understanding are the outcome of reflection. We need a lot of it, since, in psychiatry, meaning and understanding are so constantly corrupted by the impact of psychosis.

'Reflection' demands taking a long, hard look at what we do, and how well we are doing it. It might be called 'audit', but the audit includes unconscious aspects of the service and its functioning. We need this mirror on a fairly frequent basis. At the most detailed level of a team's work, there is always a job to be done on assessing how well the job is being done, how well things are going, how well a patient is doing, and how effective a piece of work is. We need to take stock of how the hopes of success drift away from the reality of small improvements. Our hopes of ourselves need to stay within reach of what is practical.

There is a second reason for reflection. The capacity of psychotic patients to preserve that function for themselves is woefully small and erratic at best. Inevitably, the staff are recruited to be the patients' capacity to respect reality, just as their self-care and self-knowledge are transferred to staff for safe keeping.

Because reflection and meaning-generation are significant elements of both therapy and staff support, there is a risk of confusing reflection on the work with a therapeutic reflection on oneself. That confusion is understandable, but the boundary needs to be kept. It is a corruption of the task of reflection in a work organisation if it drifts too much into an apparent therapy of the staff. Clarity of purpose is important. Staff need to collect their minds for *reflection on the work*, and their experience of, and reactions to it. In particular, the team needs time to address its performance over even the smallest detail of the work – the hopes, in all their exaggeration, need to be put alongside the actual realistic achievements, however minute. This is the programme for staff support – to examine achievements, unrealistic hopes, and any connected experience of underachieving. A watchful eye needs to be kept on a drift into the confidence that comes from the stereotypes and invulnerability.

Reflection as counter-culture

The drift towards personalised therapy is not the only, or the main, form of corruption of self-reflection. At times, in certain institutions that care for people, reflection takes second place in the culture. Often well-advertised, and indeed amazing, technologies have a dazzling and prominent place that pushes the duller and difficult struggle for reflection and understanding into the shadows. As a result, we may have to protect reflection in the institution. It comes easily under threat from the various reactions to stress we have discussed. A space in the work activity needs to be created for enquiring in a self-reflective manner. This means more than simply setting a time for a support group. It means more than engaging an external group facilitator or consultant. It means protecting the *attitudes* that form the reflective stance. The culture itself needs to be a 'culture of enquiry' (see Main 1967; Griffiths and Hinshelwood 2001), and the attitudes need to be continually reinforced against corruption. Any support group for staff stress needs to embody and represent those attitudes. The support group represents values of honesty and reality, and should do so quite explicitly.

Listening scientifically for signs and symptoms of psychosis, in order to make an objective diagnosis and plan effective pharmaceutical and other treatments, is a particular kind of meaning. It satisfies staff, and often patients and their relatives. However, it does not imply that we abandon listening to the person in order to make sense of his experience.

Diagnostic meaning and reflective meaning need to be kept in tandem. However, listening in the mechanical and scientific manner seems in practice to restrict personal reflective listening. There is a danger here of polarising a 'scientific' form from a 'personal' reflective form of listening, and this needs clarifying (see the more extended discussion of this in 'scientific management' Essay 3, p. 145). By 'scientific' I mean categorising, quantifying and generalising what one hears, and by 'personal' I mean having an attitude of fellow-feeling, an 'I-know-how-you-feel' response to another person. As Barrett (1996) observed, the process through which each patient passes separates these functions in time: first, the 'scientific' listening does seem required by psychiatric culture, and later the personalised reinstatement of a 'moral' being (see 'Meaninglessness and understanding', p. 16). To generate meaning is the core of a mind's activity; to choose between a meaningful diagnosis and treatment on one hand and a personal understanding on the other. Meaning is something a schizophrenic's mind baulks at, and the minds of the staff must take over that function from the schizophrenic patient. In so far as this book contributes to meaningful understanding of care, it has an effect of its own – just by being read. The psychiatric job itself involves the task of keeping things meaningful. The question seems to be: 'What sort of meaning?' The answer really should be 'Both sorts'. However, a competition between psychiatric diagnosis and personal experience makes exclusive rivals of these functions.

The external consultant

The closing-off of a reflective form of understanding can often be part of the particular characteristic of caring for schizophrenic patients who do intrude on personal reflection with their invasive forms of communication. The job of keeping good reflection going is particularly difficult in psychiatry. Teams of psychiatric staff often engage consultants for regular, maybe weekly, meetings (e.g. Obholzer and Roberts 1994). (Note that the term 'consultant' means someone who leads a team to discuss their own issues. It is not to be confused with the senior medical grade in British hospitals.) This is an intuitive recognition that psychiatric teams need to reflect on their work, and should have this need provided for. Because the psychiatric task is so beset by forces against meaning and reflection, it is necessary to plan reflection as a part of the job. A consultant from outside the team is usually engaged because it is assumed that he will tend to remain clearer in mind. We must remember, though, that often a consultant who comes for a longish period begins to identify with the team – as *their* consultant – and is slowly incorporated emotionally, thus clouding his perception. Part of reflection is the process of clearing our minds. We need to clear them from the intrusion into us of our patients' anti-reflective minds. Another distortion of consultancy is that as a designated expert, a consultant can be left to do too much meaning-creation himself, when mere questions will do. The carers have dumped the difficult job of reflection solely onto him.

Assigning the role of someone from outside recognises the importance of reflecting from a distance. The 'outside' perspective implies that it will add something that cannot be found so clearly on the inside. That 'something' is the clearer capacity to make sense of the team's and the individual's experience in the work. It is as if there is a problem in having an experience and at the same time making sense of it: indeed, there is a problem. It is always difficult to find the capacity to reflect on something while it is happening to you. It is easier after the event. The external consultant, and the structure of a special meeting as time out from the face-to-face cut-and-thrust of the work, do mean that a separation is being made between the experience of doing the work, and reflecting on that experience.

An external consultant, whose presence clearly separates the functions of having an experience and of reflecting on it, is helpful, though not entirely satisfactory. The role is a resource at times, and perhaps frequently. Necessarily, it should be temporary because of the inevitable corruption of his 'outsider' status after a while. However, a second reason for the temporariness is that he can inhibit another aim – the development of an 'internal consultant'.

The internal consultant

To progress from an external consultant, the team must develop a kind of internal consultancy within the team. The crucial function is for the persons in the team to *feel understood*; so, the aim is for individual members to give that experience to each other – to understand how the others feel. Who, perhaps, could understand better than a colleague struggling with the same stress? This is something that a well-functioning team can do anyway. The role of the external consultant is therefore to enhance that sense of understanding each other, and being understood. The external consultant is often expected by the team to understand them, and thus to be the *source* of feeling understood. But so far as it is possible, he should be helping the team on the path to performing this understanding for each other.

In turn, interpersonal understanding can lead each person to understand their own individual struggles with the work – an internal understanding. That means enhancing the self-reflective capacity *within* each person. We might think of having a sort of consultant inside each person, as their own internal consultant. The individual team member has at times to think in a quite self-conscious way about making sense of her experience, as if she were talking to a small consultant hidden inside her being.

So, the overall aim is a movement: first, understanding by the external consultant; then understanding by team members of each other; and finally understanding by an individual member of herself.

The ability to inhabit that dual position – to have an experience and to give it meaning – is the core of having a human mind. That this is so difficult in psychiatric work is inherent in the work itself. It means that reflection should be especially supported. It needs to be the essence of an institution dedicated to healing minds. Precisely because of the mentally intrusive quality of the work with damaged minds, it is especially difficult to sustain self-reflection while on the job. The degree to which an individual, or a team, can do this will vary considerably. It will be partly to do with the personalities involved, but it will also depend on the emotional context in which the team is working. High levels of staff turnover, for instance, will make it much, much more difficult, since the pervading air of instability unsettles everyone, and encroaches on that internal dialogue. Making sense of the distracting instability of a team environment detracts from the energy for making sense of the reality of a particular patient, and so on.

This does not mean that everyone must be a psychoanalyst, or have psychoanalysis. It means maximising in everyone this function that makes us uniquely human. Because the pressure and the stress of the impact of the psychosis tend to subvert our human quality, a great deal of effort is needed to protect a self-reflective space within the individuals and within the team. Given the job that psychiatry is, special provision must always be made.

Essay 2

What's it like?

Psychoanalytic theories of schizophrenia

> he is an alien, a stranger, signalling to us from the void in which he is foundering, a void which may be peopled by presences that we do not even dream of. They used to be called demons and spirits, and they used to be known and named. He has lost his sense of self, his feelings, his place in the world as we know it. He tells us he is dead.
>
> (Laing 1967, p. 110)

This essay asks what is the impact of psychosis on the sufferer. There are various accounts by psychiatrists, by novelists and by the sufferers of what it is like (e.g. Green 1964; Kesey 1962; Frame 1962; Read 1989, Berke *et al.* 2002). Psychoanalysts have closely studied many clinical cases and treatments (e.g. Heimann 1942; Segal 1950; Rosenfeld 1965; Sechehaye 1951; Sohn 1995; Sinason 1993; Conran 1999; Jackson 2001). They all reveal the agony experienced, and often deflected. Psychoanalytic treatment for psychosis is difficult to practise and requires extensive training, supervision, experience, and support. It cannot be a routine treatment.

Because of this, some argue that psychoanalysis has no part to play in psychiatry. Indeed, some general psychiatrists view psychoanalysis with disapproval or worse. Modern methods of visualising the brain and its functions, and research into global and localised synapse physiology, have seemingly sidelined psychoanalysis. It is said to be resistant to the kind of empirical verification that constitutes a scientific evidence-base as currently defined, and is believed to have no empirical methods comparable to those used on the material brain. (Drug treatments have a demonstrated effectiveness, but on their own terms (see Essay 3). In addition, the commercial success of drugs has for five decades or so made considerable sums of money available for the advertising and promotion of pharmaceutical treatments. This has created a climate of expectation that drugs are the natural treatment of choice. Moreover, this promotional activity has created an expectation that the drug trial is the natural research method for assessing effectiveness.)

Even among psychoanalysts there is dispute about the extent to which psychotic patients have benefited from psychoanalytic discoveries, and whether they have been properly evidenced (Willick 2001). Lucas (2003) has stoutly defended a psychoanalytic enquiry that reveals the meanings of bizarre symptoms and experiences. Not only does that understanding fit with what the patient is looking for, but psychoanalytically oriented formulation is important in the management of cases (Lucas 2003), and in assessing someone's suitability for psychotherapy (Alanen *et al.* 1991, Jackson and Williams 1994; see for instance the overview by Reilly (1997). The Arbours Association also practises a mixed psychotherapy and physical therapy treatment (Berke *et al.* 2002)). The Nordic system of needs-adapted psychiatry (Cullberg 2001) demonstrated convincing possibilities for the selective use of psychoanalytically oriented therapy as part of a general psychosis service.

Curiously, feelings in professional debate can become heated about the place of psychoanalysis (see 'Treatment choices' in Essay 3, p. 138). As much as anything these are ideological points of view, and it is important not to counter ideology with a counter-ideology. Instead, we need to attend to co-operative ventures that respect bio-medical and psychoanalytic (and other) therapies. Jones (1929) long ago called (obviously in vain) for such a mutual respect. Indeed, Freud (1917c) in a similar discussion, dwelt on the precise differences and competitiveness between psychoanalysis and psychiatry, concluding that the relations should be 'one supplementing the other' (Freud 1917c, p. 254; see 'Psychiatry and psychoanalysis' in Essay 3, p. 124). Combining psychopharmacology and therapeutic endeavour *in practice* significantly improves recoveries and sustains improvement. Grotstein (2001, p. 17) acknowledges the relevance of the research literature on the physical basis of psychosis, while assigning to psychoanalysis and psychoanalytic psychotherapy the equally relevant role of 'assistance in and restoration of their capacity to find meaning in their fractionated thinking'.

In short, the place for psychoanalysis in understanding the psychology of psychosis, and enriching psychiatric services, is probably extensive, although the direct use of psychoanalytic treatment is probably limited.

Dimensions of understanding

Psychoanalytic understanding of schizophrenia is based entirely on the reflective form as described in Essay 1 ('Reflective practice', p. 38). However, there are subjective features that occur with regularity in the experiences of psychotic people, allowing some generalisation of their subjectivity. These regular features are:

- turning away from the real world;
- a self-absorption that makes one's imaginings real;
- the cognitive loosening of links between thoughts;
- the loss of abstraction and symbolisation;
- missing the sense of a consistent self.

Recognising these regular features is not so different from the approach used in diagnostic psychiatry, where, however, the priority is to render these experiences into an objective form, apparent to an external observer (the psychiatrist) and quantifiable across a selected population. Our attention here is directed more to the way psychosis can be understood than to how it can be psychologically cured.

The general features crop up with varying emphasis in most psychoanalytic accounts, and give rise to a number of dimensions that may overlap or may be orthogonal, as follows:

- *Classical symptoms*: Delusions, hallucinations, emotional flatness, identity confusions, and cognitive deficits are seen as
  - primary, i.e. the symptoms directly represent the process itself;
  - secondary, arising in compensation to the underlying psychotic process.
- *Causal factors*: Different psychoanalytic theories attribute the specific psychotic problems to widely varying sets of causal factors. These factors are divided into
  - *intra-psychic* ones, which may be
    - those that focus on the interpretation of symbols, much as Freud did with his neurotic patients;

    - those that theorise a deeper problem in the formation and use of symbols themselves
  - *environmental factors* (referring to the personal environment of other people), including impingements by others on the experience and identity of the patient. The emphasis may be on
    - early impingements in the infancy of the patient;
    - current dissonance arising from a lack of attunement by the analyst.
- *Psychoanalytic practice*: Even more widely varying are the methods of intervention used in practice, which may feed back into modified theory. Roughly speaking, three categories of intervention may be discerned:
  - interpretation of the unconscious;
  - attunement of analyst to patient;
  - various non-psychoanalytic interventions such as support, suggestion, education, and self-revelation (of the analyst) and so on.

Different schools also vary as to the significant aetiological causes.

- *The conflict theory* – there is an overwhelming charge of some impulse or anxiety, which takes the mind away from the real world;
- *The deficit theory* – there is a deliberate psychic act of self-harm which dismantles the capacity to recognise one's problems, and in the process dismantles many other mental functions.

The variety of features to which psychoanalysts give weight appears complex, and I shall lay out the theories in a sequence that simplifies the state of affairs somewhat, i.e.

1 theories that address the cognitive deficit primarily;
2 those that stress the dissonance between self and others;
3 those that focus on the existential problems.

Freud's starting point

Psychoanalytic approaches to psychosis originated with Freud's view that schizophrenic patients do not make a relationship with others, because they have lost interest in reality (and hence there is no transference to the analyst). As a result a plethora of theories, and their derived forms of treatment, have grown up over nearly a century to fill this gap in Freud's achievement. Freud's initial pessimism seems to have proved unfounded. Later treatment of schizophrenic patients has demonstrated that such patients do in fact make relationships.

Freud's estimate of psychotic patients was dismal:

> I did not like those patients . . . They make me angry and I find myself irritated to experience them so distant from myself and from all that is human. This is an astonishing intolerance which brands me a poor psychiatrist. (Freud in a letter to Istvan Hollos in 1928, quoted in Dupont 1988, p. 251)

Freud was troubled by that lack of being human. As always, however, what troubled him provoked his curiosity, and often when he could not make progress clinically he developed theory instead. He found psychotic patients clearly different from neurotics, who, he had found, were occupied by thoroughly human dilemmas and conflicts (Freud 1900).

Freud's work on neurosis and the unconscious was in full flood in 1906 when Carl Jung began to correspond with Freud, and a cohort, including Eugene Bleuler and colleagues, joined up from Zurich. The Zurich group were attracted to Freud because they found his discovery of the meaning of dreams a useful method by which to approach the meaning of psychotic patients' utterances. The Zurich group had been influenced by Jung's 'word association test' (Jung 1906) as a means of touching on underlying complexes that distorted mental associations. Both Jung and Freud, as well as Janet and many other clinicians at the turn of the century, were using the conceptual framework of associationist psychology as it had passed down from Locke in the seventeenth century. Jung and Freud held the view that mental illnesses were to do with specific abnormal associations in the mind, complexes of mental contents, which were inappropriately aggregated together. This contrasted with most other psychologists of the time, who believed that mental disorder was to do with a loosening of associations, a lost capacity to keep mental contents together.

For the Zurich group, dreams represented another means of accessing these complexes, and perhaps a means of giving more specific content to them.[1] At the time, Freud was developing his notion of transference.[2] At the moment when Freud was concentrating on the meanings and importance of transference he was confronted with enthusiastic colleagues who wanted to tell him about their work with psychotics. Bleuler, for instance, invented the term 'schizophrenia' (Bleuler 1911). In the inevitably rivalrous situation with colleagues who were heading in the same direction, Freud must have felt somewhat at a disadvantage. He could not use his own developing method as it was moving towards an emphasis on transference, and a transference relationship was exactly what Freud found missing with psychotic patients. Freud could not debate with his new Zurich colleagues on their specific interest.

To enter this new domain Freud had to move in another direction. When eventually he could find that direction, he had already parted company with Jung.[3] However, in the meantime, to keep pace with Jung and his mentor Bleuler, Freud made an initial attempt to understand psychosis through the case of Judge Schreber (Freud 1911a).

Freud and Schreber

Because psychotic patients found it difficult, or impossible, to relate to Freud, he 'analysed' Schreber's published memoirs rather than the patient, his dreams and free associations (Schreber 1903). Freud recognised that Schreber had suffered some kind of psychic upheaval experienced as a 'world catastrophe'. Schreber believed that the

1 Both Jung and Freud were working in a context where the unconscious was known about (Ellenberger 1974, Whyte 1978; and see for instance Butler 1880). What they were all doing was to try to understand how this mental unconscious worked. A comparison of the precise views of Jung, Freud and the dissociationsists (Janet 1892, Myers 1903, etc.) would be very profitable in locating their differences in the context of the time.

2 Dora (Freud 1905), a patient who had walked out on Freud in the middle of his best efforts to interpret the meanings of her dreams, did so, it seemed, because Freud represented something vitally important (and threatening) to her. He had neglected the meaning she had transferred onto him.

3 Freud's new ideas led to a whole new development in psychoanalytic theorising which enriched the work with neurotics and gave a purchase to the understanding of human nature itself. That new direction led to the theory of narcissism (Freud 1914) and the paper on mourning and melancholia (Freud 1917a). It involved a turn towards an emphasis on the object of the instinct (hence object-relations theory), in contrast to psychic energy and the economic model of the mind.

world had come to an end. His ensuing delusions were then, according to Freud, an attempt at reconstructing a world to live in. Significantly, the central core of Schreber's delusional system was a belief that God required Schreber to repopulate the world after the catastrophe, and to do so from his own body as if he were a woman. This regeneration came *after* the catastrophe and pointed Freud to his two-phase view of psychosis – first, a psychic catastrophe (the breakdown proper), and then a reconstruction creating a world of delusions and hallucinations.

Freud's analysis of the case diverged from his normal approach with neurotics, whereby he tracked down a conflict. With Schreber, he needed to explain the world catastrophe, the primary event in the illness. He saw this as differing from repression, the core of neurosis. The psychotic obliterates his conflict in a completely different way. Freud's term was 'disavowal'. He used his economic model of the way psychic energy circulates, and his notion of cathexis is important here – cathexis means the investment of interest and attention (libido) in some particular object. That is, the libido is turned towards an object (invests it), thus giving that object special interest or importance. The Freudian paradigm is falling in love with a sexual partner; the object of affection becomes of supreme interest, as she/he is invested with great importance to the lover. That interest that invests something or someone is, in Freud's model, psychic energy. Psychic energy is instinctual, and is typically the energy of the libido. The greater the amount of the libido that is invested, the greater the fascination.

In repression, the libido attaches to some important unconscious memory, but in consciousness, the libido is directed instead towards some substitute object or idea. A spider is made to substitute for a poisonous entangling version of a mother (for instance). Here, the cathexis of the mother is removed because she arouses the hate inherent in frustration. Instead, as a direct substitute, a spider is cathected – libido is directed towards the spider instead of the mother.

In psychosis the energy involved in the actual real world reduces to zero, leaving the person with no object of interest or fascination. He disavows the existence of anything worth directing his libido towards. The libido is withdrawn altogether from everything outside the patient. Hence the actual world loses all its interest. It is a 'catastrophe' to the external world, as the patient experiences it. It does not mean anything to him any more. Involved in that catastrophe are the persons in the actual world, who become of no interest either. Thus the psychotic seems not to relate to others, not even a well-meaning analyst such as Freud. This was the difficulty Freud found, and disavowal (withdrawal of libido, in contrast to a substitute object in repression) was his method of explaining the difficulty.

As clinical experience was lacking, Freud concentrated on theoretical aspects of the instinctual drives. Although he did concern himself with interpreting the symbolic meanings of Schreber's delusions, without dreams and associations he was on less sure ground. Of course he was driven to this for technical reasons; he did not have the associations with which he could trace the hidden symbolic meanings in the way he analysed dreams. He had no possibility of making interpretations to the patient. He could not gain validity for his interpretations by curing Schreber. Nevertheless, Freud believed that Schreber's delusions held traces of what had happened to his mind, and why. He noted the importance of men to Schreber, particularly the male doctors. Associated with them was the 'male' God which Schreber felt was behind all his problems. (We now know that Schreber was in fact brought up by a father who had achieved wide fame for his views on the upbringing of children in which the child is reduced to extreme passivity in metal and leather harnesses to promote correct posture (Schreber 1903 (1955 edn), Schatzman 1973, Shengold 1989; and see 'Science as cultural attitudes' in Essay 3, p. 132).) Moreover, Schreber believed that the world after the catastrophe was to be reconstituted with a whole new race of beings, and that they would be procreated through his own body. Schreber believed that he was chosen by God to effect this repopulation, and to this end his own body was being turned into a female one. Freud's view of these beliefs – the importance of male persons, the use of his body for procreation, and his transmutation into a woman – pointed to homosexual impulses. It seemed that the horror of finding himself a homosexual was so catastrophic to Schreber that it literally blew his mind. Instead of finding substitutes for his homosexual impulses, Schreber's mind was completely reorganised in order to create a delusional order – a homosexual one. Schreber's homosexuality was expressed quite differently from that of a neurotic. He literally lived the belief that homosexuality was forced upon him; moreover, he sustained his self-esteem by ascending to a position of supreme importance – Schreber himself would be the begetter of the new world brought into existence after the catastrophe. His homosexuality was not relegated to the unconscious domain; it became the principle for reconstituting a new – though delusional – world repopulated by him.

At the time that Freud was struggling with psychosis in the form of Schreber's memoirs, he was also writing his paper on 'Two principles of mental functioning' (Freud 1911b), in which he formulated the pleasure principle and the reality principle. In the normal development of an infant, the awareness of reality begins to put a check on a child's demand for immediate satisfactions (the pleasure from satisfied instinctual needs). A kind of truce develops in the contest between its demands and the reality of the parents' attentions. Pleasure and demandingness are partially limited. However, his theory of the Schreber case is that under certain circumstances, the reality principle is overthrown by a withdrawal of interest in, or cathexis of, the real world of others, and the parents or carers who represent limits. This formulation of a reality principle arose in conjunction with his understanding of Schreber. Precisely how the reality principle was compromised in a psychotic was only worked out later (Freud 1915, 1924a, 1924b). In general, cathexis is turned away from the real world, which has then lost all meaning. In contrast, the neurotic retains meaning in the external world, which the psychotic gives up.

This does not mean that the psychotic is completely oblivious to the real world: he still understands that if he is hungry he needs to eat food, and will do so when he has the chance. Instead, it means that such a natural connection for most of us becomes a meaningless activity. The whole set of significances in the real world is diminished, and to all intents and purposes lost, for the psychotic. The libido, having turned away from the actual external world, turns towards the ego itself. As a result, the person becomes the centre of all interest: a state of narcissism (Freud 1914). The psychotic is for Freud the great exemplar of narcissism, and this suggested to him that he call the psychoses the 'narcissistic neuroses'. In the narcissistic state, the ego reverts to itself as the loved object, and hence his own productions, phantasies, are prized above the external world and supersede reality as delusions and hallucinations. It is a solipsistic self-centred world. The libido shifts from a focus outside (on objects) to a focus within (on the ego). Therefore, Freud concluded (1914), the libido has two interchangeable forms: object-libido and ego-libido.

In his early work on dreams, Freud (1900) considered the correspondence between dreams and insanity. In sleep, the scene of a dream is experienced as reality, as real as the hallucinations of psychotic people. There was some process by which the products of the mind could come to be experienced as if they were real perceptions. The *déjà vu* experience that quite normal people have, but in a waking state, is an example of a pseudo-real experience that we all know. Freud postulated that there was an abnormal distribution of psychic energy. Some psychic energy is habitually directed, as one's attention, towards perception (or rather towards what is revealed in perception – the contents of the visual field, for instance). However, in the specific states of dreaming and hallucinating, that energy moves towards memories and phantasies, giving them the status of objective reality. Only after the Schreber case was this hypothesis elaborated and superseded.

Freud's conclusions from the Schreber case are not all of equal significance. His view that all psychosis is related to unacceptable homosexual impulses has hardly stood the test of time. However, two theoretical conclusions have led to important developments in psychoanalytic knowledge: the theory of narcissism (Freud 1914), and the theory of the reality principle (Freud 1911b).

Psychosis and symbolism

Freud had formed psychoanalysis on the neurotic problem of symbolisation. Something repressed in the unconscious comes to be represented by other elements of reality. They are substitutes, and are useful precisely because they are substitutes and can disguise the original thing they substitute for. They keep the unconscious element unrecognised. This is the story of dreams as Freud told it (Freud 1900). However, Freud realised that symbolisation in psychosis was of a completely different order.

In his 1915 essay on the unconscious, Freud put the evidence for and nature of the unconscious on a systematic and theoretical basis. Part of that was to distinguish it from the preconscious (and consciousness). He located the psychotic problem at the heart of that distinction. Normally, he argued, the contents of the preconscious are those of the unconscious that had been tamed, as it were, by being brought into contact with words. An object can be presented to the preconscious, and therefore consciousness, when it is a combination of a 'thing-presentation' (raw sense data) and its appropriate 'word-presentation'. Some active process occurs to combine the perceptual data with a symbolic form (typically words). The result of the combination is a presentation capable of being conscious – an 'object-presentation'.

Then in psychosis some abnormality occurs in the process so the unconscious thing-presentations (not available to consciousness) become modified in a different way. There is not a normal combination. The distinction between 'thing' and 'word' is lost. Words get treated like things even in conscious utterances. Freud suggested that in the first phase, the world catastrophe, the libido withdraws, and decathects the presentations of outer things; then, in the second phase, there is a recathexis of words – as things.

Thing-presentations in the unconscious coexist with object-presentations in the preconscious and conscious. The two domains deal with their contents according to different rules. In the unconscious, the primary process consists largely of condensation and displacement; whereas in the preconscious, the contents are dealt with by the ordinary processes of rational thought, involving the rules of semantics, signs and logic. So, the primary process is the set of rules for thing-presentations, as in dreams; the secondary process rules the objects of consciousness. In psychosis, therefore, the reversion of words to things accords with the very concrete way in which schizophrenics use words. It also explains how a schizophrenic's conscious thinking often appears to resemble the primary process of a dream. In neurosis, conscious mental contents retain their symbolic quality, but not in psychosis.

Because of his breakthrough in understanding dreams and the way their symbolism works, Freud was drawn to an explanation of psychosis that would also depend on symbols. Sticking to the field of symbol-formation led Freud to see psychosis as an abnormality of the very formation of symbols, while neurosis involves abnormal ways of using symbols that have been formed properly.

Sadly, by the time that Freud had fully worked through all these ideas in 1915, he and Jung had gone their separate ways. Freud's complex theory could no longer play a part in the Freud–Jung collaboration and rivalry. It was, however, important as a radical development in understanding psychosis and in taking psychoanalytic theory forward from its early years as a theory of sexuality and dreams. Despite the ingenuity of this theory, it seems that Freud found little use for it. He still didn't know how to treat psychosis.

Schizophrenia and perception

When Freud returned to the problem of psychosis in 1924, his excitement at the theoretical possibilities of the structural model (described in 1923) replaced his interest in his topographical formulation. Freud's theory of the super-ego brought in a new conception of the schizophrenic's problem. His 1923 paper was a crucial landmark that described a much enriched theory of the agencies of mind. This 'structural model' of the id, ego and super-ego immediately showed its importance as an advanced tool for understanding clinical phenomena. One year afterwards, he returned to an explanation of the reality problem in psychosis (Freud 1924a, 1924b). His two short papers still owe more to theoretical enthusiasm than to clinical cases.

He started in the first paper (Freud 1924a) with the abstract observation that in both neurosis and psychosis there is a conflict between the id and external reality. The neurotic ego breaks away from the id, the instinctual impulses being repudiated and repressed because they do not conform to the expectations of the external world of other people. The same balancing act – between id impulses and external reality – leads the psychotic ego to ally itself with the id and to back away from reality, thus to 'disavow' the external world. There is a pleasing neatness about this paradigm. However, it is not without problems. Neurotics also distort reality, but they do it in a different way. He attempted then to understand the different distortions of reality made by the neurotic and by the psychotic (Freud 1924b). Neurosis, like psychosis, has two stages, he argued. In the neurotic, an id impulse towards an object in the external world is repressed, but only imperfectly, and in a second stage the impulse returns and attaches to another, inappropriate, object. In this way, the neurotic distorts the relations with that substitute object, which is then dealt with symbolically by phobic flight, obsessive control, etc. The spider can be avoided instead of the phantasy persecutor. In psychosis, on the other hand, reality is damaged in stage one. It is disavowed, leaving as it were a gap in the appreciation of reality altogether. In the second stage that gap is covered over, as if with a bandage, by an invented reality. So, in neurosis, reality is distorted in the second stage; in psychosis it is given up in the first stage.

The developing ideas

In summary, Freud made a number of conjectures about the disorder at the root of psychosis. Some were more grounded in empirical findings than others, but overall he was postulating the malfunction of processes that he had discovered in neurotic patients. We have seen the four main hypotheses he put forward.

1. Psychic energy reverts (regresses) from the perceptual apparatus towards memory and phantasy, giving them the quality of reality.
2. The libido withdraws from, and abandons, external reality, invests the attention in the person's own thoughts and feelings, and creates a replacement world of personal delusions and hallucinations.
3. There is a collapse of the distinction between things and words, so that words become things, and proper symbols and representations cannot be formed or used.
4. Because of an intolerable conflict between the id and reality, the ego abandons reality – in contrast to the neurotic, who represses reality and uses inappropriate substitute objects (still in reality).

Freud's idea that something happens to symbols (words) so that they become concrete things for the schizophrenic mind has been followed up in many ways. It offered a way into the precise process of the very severe cognitive loss in schizophrenia.

All the later psychoanalytic views on psychosis derive from some aspects of Freud's work: symbolism, narcissism, the reality principle and specific defence mechanisms. The later theories cluster around several dimensions, which I will deal with as: symbol formation; psychotic and non-psychotic parts of the personality; primary process and ego-weakness; omnipotence and identity; the existential problem; and interpersonal relations.

Symbol formation

Melanie Klein, among other psychoanalysts, respected Freud's hypothesis that the schizophrenic's cognitive deficit can be traced to some abnormality in the development of symbol use. When a four-year-old boy, Dick, appeared completely unable to form and use symbols, she traced the problem back to very intense aggression and fear.

On the basis of her work with children, she had moved her emphasis from sexuality to destructiveness. The Oedipus complex is as much to do with aggression as with sex. Oedipus killed his father. He was a murderer – as well as being occupied with sex and incest. Moving psychoanalytic attention from sexuality to aggression did actually follow one of Freud's ideas – that in depression a person hates herself for being hateful (Freud 1917a). Some can rationalise their hate as thoroughly justifiable, and thus idealise their aggression. Others subside into self-reproach and self-loathing – clinical depression. A phobic patient may identify her aggression as externalised in the form of a spider, say, and run away from it. Or an obsessional may spend hours turning off gas-taps or locking the doors, and in some such symbolic way, shut off their own aggressive impulses. Such neurotic symptoms are devoted to controlling impulses – and they could theoretically control sexual ones as much as aggressive ones. But in terms of the more severe disturbances – psychoses – Klein proposed that the conflict over aggressive impulses is much more intense than with sexual ones.

Her patient Dick (Klein 1930) lost his own ability to symbolise and to think. She thought that this happened as a failure of repression. She had noticed that one way in which a child dealt with its aggression towards important people was to find a substitute object, whereby the ambivalence of needing and hating could be diminished by turning to a new, unblemished person. Thus a child might transfer affection away from mother and towards a schoolmistress, in order to deal with frustrations, threats and concerns in the relation with mother. (Ultimately a little boy will move from mother to find a substitute eventually in a wife – a process that Freud demonstrated in the Little Hans case (Freud 1909a).) Klein saw this as one imperative for finding and using symbols: they could act as similar substitute objects. Toys are a very good example whereby ambivalence, violence and hopeless remorse can be played out away from the vitally needed parents.

Dick had almost lost the capacity for using symbols – on which, of course, Klein's method of child analysis depended. He did not play with toys, and appeared indifferent to all the stimuli that normally arouse a child's interest. He seemed interested only in door handles. He was very active and not inhibited in the ordinary sense. He ran about, but in a mindless way, and occasionally would hide himself in the gap between the double doors of the play room. It was clear to her that this was a psychotic boy who had taken a more or less completely different developmental path from the normal one. It was qualitatively different from the neurotic, and dream use of symbols. Dick couldn't form symbols at all. He was inhibited from this because the normal process of finding a substitute object failed him. His aggression was so extreme that even finding a substitute object to love in a protected enclave away from his aggression just did not work. His aggression pervaded everything. So, with no powers of substitution he had no symbols, and no cognitive development could occur.

Like Freud, Klein thought that the failure to form symbols indicated psychosis rather than neurosis. Dick's whole life seemed to be one of restricted ability to symbolise or represent his world meaningfully to himself. (In fact, he did not resemble the ordinary child schizophrenic, as he did not use symbols for creating delusions and hallucinations either. The picture is one that we might now recognise as autism. Childhood autism was not described as a syndrome until Kanner's description in 1943.) Through her understanding of the extreme violence, her interpretations did engender the resumption of some symbol development in the boy. In the process she was impressed that development involved the replacement of indifference with intense and specific anxieties. He became a more anxious boy but a more normal one, a boy who could begin to represent and symbolise his anxieties.

The clinical picture in this report by Klein appeared to represent the first stage of the psychotic process as described by Freud. There was an actual obliteration of the symbolic world and of any representations. The boy had achieved an indifference to external reality; its meaning for him did not exist (it had perhaps been catastrophically lost). What Dick did not show was the second phase that Freud described in the Schreber case. Dick did not reconstruct a meaningful world to cover the gap in the real external world.

Psychosis here seems to be a failure of symbol formation to develop, but later Klein began to notice different processes (Klein 1946). She began to hypothesise that in psychosis, the hate for oneself takes the form of actual self-directed aggression, and leads to self-destructive phenomena: horrendous forms of suicide, self-mutilations, and more subtle destructive processes that have damaging effects on the persons' own minds. Freud had speculated that the core of the psychotic process was to withdraw the libido and to direct it narcissistically towards the ego, towards the self; Klein followed an analogous conceptual path, but she worked with the possibility that the ego withdrew aggression from objects in the external world to redirect it, 'narcissistically', against itself. Later Kleinians (e.g. Rosenfeld 1971) would term these self-directed negative impulses 'negative narcissism'. These processes involved a specific dismantling of ego-capacities, especially the loss of the ability to have certain feelings – often violent feelings (Klein 1946). She described this as a self-destructive process. Parts of the ego could simply go out of existence, and she described how she could watch this in the course of a session, often with a subsequent return of these experiences that had been annihilated. She called this active process of dividing off parts of the ego 'splitting of the ego', a schizoid defence, and thus one of the core elements of schizophrenia.

Klein (1946) thought that the deepest and perhaps the earliest anxiety the ego has to deal with is the experience that the coherence of the mind is in itself in jeopardy. She believed that this is the direct effect of the death instinct. The breaking up of the ego must inevitably result in a serious hole in understanding reality: both the real world and the world of personal impulses inside the person (i.e. a retreat from both external and internal realities). This leads to the serious cognitive deficits in schizophrenia. There is here a severe loss of the capacity to know about aspects of the self that have been split apart, and indeed a corruption of a sense of knowing who one is, i.e. one's sense of identity.

To pursue this Kleinian line, we must move to the work of Klein's students in the 1950s when they built on the ideas in these papers (Klein 1930, 1946) by analysing schizophrenic patients. Wilfred Bion developed with Hanna Segal (1957) and others (Rosenfeld 1965) Klein's ideas on the nature of language and symbolic thinking as revealed by investigating cognitive abnormalities in schizophrenia (Bion 1959, 1962a). In his key paper, Bion (1957) returned to Freud's investigation of the loss of reality.

Psychotic and non-psychotic parts of the mind

One of Freud's observations in the Schreber case was that late in the illness the patient was able to converse in perfectly ordinary ways, appropriate to his status as an appeal court judge, while at the same time he harboured delusions and his belief in his reconstructed and repopulated world. Schreber could conduct himself quite appropriately when invited to the dinner table of the medical superintendent and could discourse upon the affairs of the world in a thoroughly intelligent way, while his bizarre delusional system remained at bay. A passage from Freud (1940) much later is little noticed but suggests that a reality-oriented part of the schizophrenic's mind survives continuously through the psychotic bouts:

> One learns from patients after their recovery that at the time in some corner of their mind (as they put it) there was a normal person hidden, who, like a detached spectator, watched the hubbub of illness go past him. (Freud 1940, p. 202).

In fact this notion of a sane part of the person existing alongside the mad goes back to Breuer and his patient, Anna O: 'a clear-sighted and calm observer sat, as she put it, in a corner of her brain and looked on at all the mad business' (Breuer and Freud 1895, p. 46).

In Freud's economic terms, some part of the ego remains connected to the actual external world – reality is at least partly cathected. However, there is a sense of a structural arrangement – separate 'persons', normal and psychotic, inside the patient.

In 1953 a symposium on the theory of schizophrenia was held at the 18th International Psycho-Analytical Congress in London. Moritz Katan (1954) introduced the notion of the non-psychotic part of the personality of psychotic patients. He postulated, like Freud, that schizophrenic symptoms are an attempt at restitution, and thus the pre-psychotic phase is the important driving force. Katan believed that the pre-psychotic conflict is one focused on a narcissistic form of the Oedipus complex. The Oedipus complex is solved by breaking with reality. But he observed with surprise that the pre-psychotic conflict does persist, although it 'does not remain constant in size but changes all the time. It increases and decreases in size continually' (Katan 1954, p. 126).

Bion gave a paper at the same symposium (Bion 1954). He must surely have been struck by the idea of psychotic and non-psychotic parts of the mind coexisting, because he gave his own thoughts on just that topic in a paper to the British Psychoanalytical Society two years later, in 1955. That paper was on differentiating the psychotic from the non-psychotic parts of the personality (Bion 1957). He did not follow Katan's formulation. His interest, like Freud's, focused attention on the development and vicissitudes of the reality principle in schizophrenics. He referred to Freud's paper on 'the two principles of mental functioning' (Freud 1911b), and concentrated on the ego's reality-based function.

> I assume that when Freud speaks of the ego's allegiance to reality he is speaking of the developments he described as taking place within the institution of the reality principle . . . he said, 'the new demands made a succession of adaptations necessary in the mental apparatus, which, on account of insufficient knowledge, we can only detail very cursorily'. He then lists: the heightened significance of the sense organs directed towards the outer world and of the consciousness attached to them; attention, which he calls a special function, which had to search the outer world in order that its data might be already familiar if an urgent need should arise; a system of notation whose task was to deposit the results of this periodical activity of consciousness which he describes as a part of that which we call memory; judgement which had to decide whether a particular idea was true or false; the employment of motor discharge in appropriate alteration of reality and not simply in unburdening the mental apparatus of accretions of stimuli; and finally thought which he says made it possible to tolerate the frustration which is an inevitable accompaniment of action by virtue of its quality as an experimental way of acting. (Bion 1957, pp. 45–46)

These functions of the ego, which comprise the reality principle, are Bion's starting point. He attributed the failure of these functions to develop properly to a hatred of reality, with the result that:

> the psychotic splits his objects, and contemporaneously all that part of his personality, which would make him aware of the reality he hates, into exceedingly small fragments. (Bion 1957, p. 47)

Bion went on to say that all the functions that make up the reality principle are attacked in the same sadistic way by this self-destructive force 'and then expelled from the personality to penetrate, or encyst, the objects' (Bion 1957, p. 47). In this, Bion was armed with Klein's theory concerning aggression turned back to the self, resulting in splitting of the ego (Klein 1946). The ego destroys its own capacity to link with reality, that link being perception. Therefore, the ego's self-mutilation of its own roots, the perceptual capacities, could be viewed as a manifestation of death instinct:

> Such is the dominance of this phantasy that it is evident that it is

> no phantasy, but a fact, to the patient, who acts as if his perceptual apparatus could be split into minute fragments and projected into his objects. (Bion 1957, pp. 46–47)

Thus, a psychotic projects those parts of himself which were once concerned with perceiving things. For instance, 'If the piece of the personality is concerned with sight, the gramophone when played is felt to be watching the patient' (p. 48). Reality is not therefore completely forsaken, since it is now composed of bizarre representations of this kind. It is reconstructed, and repopulated with parts of the ego itself.

Bion also asserted that this complex psychotic process is never complete; rather 'that the contact with reality is masked by the dominance, in the patient's mind and behaviour, of an omnipotent phantasy that is intended to destroy either reality or the awareness of it' (p. 46). So, a more normal, or 'neurotic', part of the mind is concealed and overlaid by this psychotic 'phantasy' about reality. The psychotic phantasy says that reality either won't exist or will not be perceived, while the neurotic says that reality does exist but turns its back. So, the non-psychotic part of the personality resorts to repression, but the psychotic part of the personality gets rid of the apparatus on which the psyche depends to carry out the repressions. As a result:

> The non-psychotic personality was concerned with a neurotic problem, that is to say a problem that centred on the resolution of a conflict of ideas and emotions to which the operation of the ego had given rise. But the psychotic personality was concerned with the problem of repair of the ego. (Bion 1957, p. 57).

Representation and 'alpha-function'

Later, Bion (1962b) elaborated this model of the psychotic functioning mind. Like Freud, he understood that there was a conversion process from the raw data of external and internal reality. That is, a process occurs that prevents raw sense impressions from being expelled, and delivers them up to the functions of a maturing mind. Those functions that comprise the reality principle form a process that he named 'alpha-function':

> The more general statement of the theory is this: To learn from

> experience alpha-function must operate on the awareness of emotional experience; alpha-elements are produced from the impressions of the experience; these are thus made storable and available for dream thoughts and for unconscious waking thinking. (Bion 1962b, p. 8)

This does not coincide with Freud's (1915) process. Raw data in the unconscious become attached to words – making object-presentations. Bion does not make reference to Freud's description of the process, and his views diverge sharply at this point.

When he wrote the Schreber 'case study', Freud was impressed by the form of thinking that underlay Schreber's delusions, and its contrast to normal thinking. Freud at the time seemed to equate that contrast in thinking with the primary and secondary processes that discriminate between the unconscious and conscious forms of thought. Freud therefore implied that a mind operates two distinct forms of thinking – the adhesion of word-presentations to sense impressions brings mental contents from the primary process to the rigour of secondary-process thought. Bion, however, made a different differentiation: a neurotic makes a sharp distinction between unconscious and conscious, between primary and secondary processes, but the psychotic suffers from a prior problem. The psychotic deals with sense impressions by preventing them from becoming the objects of thought at all, either conscious or unconscious. Only when sense impressions have become psychological entities can they become conscious or unconscious. A psychotic, he says, exists in a sort of limbo, neither properly conscious nor unconscious, and not subject to either primary- or secondary-process thinking. For Freud, the contents of the unconscious and preconscious can coexist, in different states and under different rules. For Bion, alpha-function converts the data from raw sense impressions to usable mental objects, conscious and unconscious. For Freud the unprocessed unconscious contents are the material of dreams, but for Bion the raw data must be processed by alpha-function in order to become 'the furniture of dreams'.

According to Bion, alpha-function fails in the psychotic and there is no proper distinction between conscious and unconscious contents. Without alpha-function, 'mental contents' tend to be an accumulation of unprocessed beta-elements, not properly mental and suitable only for expulsion.

Bion understood schizophrenia as a self-directed attack (by the death instinct) on the perceptual apparatus, specifically on alpha-function as the means of linking the perceptual apparatus to the mind through processing sense data (Bion 1959). If the schizophrenic is unable to process, by alpha-function, the raw data of experience and enable it to become experiential, his mind accumulates an increasing quantity of unprocessed data. The mind must then develop as an apparatus for the evacuation of sense impressions, rather than an apparatus for having them and thinking thoughts. Indeed, Bion thought that the accumulation of the products of processed sense data generates, or even instigates in the first place, a mind to think those thoughts. They are 'thoughts in search of a thinker' as he put it, and they supply pressure for a progressive mental development. Thought disorder in a schizophrenic arises because of the impossibility of generating usable thoughts, and the ensuing accumulation of unprocessed mental contents.

Thoughts are located within a world that represents reality, external and internal (internal reality here means the world of representations properly constituted, and not the kind of concretised presentations that Freud described). In other words, the mind that can generate thoughts enters a symbolic world, a zone in which other minds can be reached. The inability to attain thoughts in any reliable way cuts the schizophrenic off from interpersonal communication, and renders that person trapped in a narcissistic world of raw sense data – 'so distant from anything human', as Freud felt.

Alpha-function turns raw sense data into experiences; another way of putting this is that the sensations acquire meaning (Hinshelwood 2003). The destruction of alpha-function is therefore the destruction of meaning; and the schizophrenic problem is that he cannot represent meanings. Bion never properly tied up this theory of alpha-function with the separation of psychotic from non-psychotic parts of the personality. The implication is that the different parts of a person are dominated by either alpha-function or by attacks upon it; the psychotic part of the personality being dominated by attacks on alpha-function (i.e. reversal of alpha-function, as Meltzer (1978) called it), and the non-psychotic by the activity of alpha-function.

Projective identification and symbolic relations

Klein's paper on schizoid mechanisms (Klein 1946) linked the 'splitting of the ego' with another associated defence mechanism, projective identification. The phantasy of annihilating a part of the ego by splitting it off is associated with another phantasy, one in which the part of the ego that is split off actually survives in another person. That part of one person's identity becomes represented by some other person's mind in the external world. The example earlier of a patient who projects his sight into the gramophone, and then thinks that the machine is watching him, conveys this mad process. This annihilation of a part of oneself is succeeded by the experience of re-finding that ego quality, function or content, but identified as some other mind or thing. This process of exporting a part of one's own identity into someone else occurs with disastrous consequences for the schizophrenic. It causes a considerable confusion in her own sense of identity. One can say that there is a boundary violation in which she loses the sureness of a sense of who she is and who the other person is. We have seen in Essay 1 the effect this can have on carers and others.

The normal act of continual symbolisation is the core of mental activity in this set of views. It was descriptively illustrated by Segal (1957), who contrasted two forms of symbolisation – symbolic equation and symbols proper. Segal's view was based on the nature of pathological projective identification. When projective identification is intense, the boundaries between oneself and other objects becomes blurred, so that a part of oneself *is* that object; they become identical:

> One [patient] whom I will call A, was a schizophrenic in a mental hospital. He was once asked by his doctor why it was that since his illness he had stopped playing the violin. He replied with some violence: 'Why? do you expect me to masturbate in public?'
>
> Another patient, B, dreamt one night that he and a young girl were playing a violin duet. He had associations to fiddling, masturbating, etc., from which it emerged clearly that the violin represented his genital and playing the violin represented a masturbation phantasy of a relation with the girl.
>
> Here then are two patients who apparently use the same symbols in the same situation — a violin representing the male genital, and playing the violin representing masturbation. The way in which the symbols function, however, is very different. For A, the violin had become so completely equated with his genital that to touch it in public became impossible. For B, playing the violin in his waking life was an important sublimation. (Segal 1957, p. 391)

Schizophrenics were found by a number of Kleinians to operate projective identification like this with serious problems of identity. Segal found the source of the abnormal form, symbolic equation typical of schizophrenics in the use of projective identification.

Segal started with a view of the symbol as tripartite: the symbol itself, the thing symbolised, and the relationship between the two. For symbols to work properly and to enable thought, there has to be a recognition that the symbol and the thing symbolised are not the same; they cannot be equated. There has to be a steady holding of boundaries. The schizophrenic's mind operates with projective identifications as if he and his object, into which he has projected a part of himself, were not adequately bounded and distinct entities. When he wants to symbolise something in his mind, it comes to be actually equated with the symbol he uses. So, the relationship between a symbol and what it symbolises is confused and merged. One becomes the other; there is an equation. The symbol *is* the thing symbolised. This way of talking about concrete symbols equated with the thing symbolised correlates with Freud's model (thing- and word-presentation become equated), while using very different concepts to explain the same phenomenon.

Primary process and ego-weakness

In *The Interpretation of Dreams*, Freud (1900) described the rules of operation of the unconscious, which depend largely on condensation and displacement rather than the ordinary rules of reason and logic (secondary process). Freud (1917b) postulated that in the schizophrenic, hallucinations obey the same primary-process rules. Schizophrenic symptoms are essentially meaningful in this view. This symbol-interpretation approach accords with the approach of Jung:

> schizophrenic utterance and behaviour could be seen as meaningful, if only it were possible to work out what the meaning might be. This was where the technique of word association was first used. (Samuels 1989, p. 4)

The consequence is that we need to decode schizophrenic symptoms, much as we do dream images. Jung was onto this before he and Freud formally joined forces. However, as Freud moved away from this view of schizophrenia with the Schreber study, Jung also developed new views. Jung evolved his theory of archetypes, upon which he elaborated his views of schizophrenic symbols. He regarded archetypal contents of the mind as carrying an especially powerful charge, so that archetypal aspects of the unconscious overwhelm the mind. Some particular access to, and response from, the collective unconscious is potentially mind-blowing:

> The contents of the schizophrenic mind remain archetypal in tone because of the mother's failure to mediate them for her infant. (Samuels 1986, p. 135)

This point about the collective, mothering context of the developing mind bears the traces of the Jungian encounter in Britain, with Winnicott and Klein.

The psychotic problem arises in the intensity that emanates from the archetypes. The intensity of image and mythical meaning inserts itself into the schizophrenic mind and disrupts it. This tradition sees schizophrenic symbols as essentially decodable. They carry meaning like dream symbols. However, it does not give any specific distinguishing mark to the psychotic problem. The psychotic's delusions are much the same as the neurotic's substitute formations. It denies a significant distinction between neurosis and psychosis, and overlooks the possibility of a deficit in symbol formation itself. It contrasts with the view that the schizophrenic condition is a problem with finding and keeping meaning itself.

Synthetic function and ego-weakness

In the ego-psychology tradition, schizophrenic symptoms can be decoded as expressions resulting from primary- rather than secondary-process thought. For instance, 'the dream exhibits all the characteristics of a psychosis' (Nunberg 1950, p. 239), the dream being an exemplar of unconscious primary process. However, how does the unconscious primary process become a conscious primary process? Ego-psychologists pay less attention to Freud's theory of thing- and word-presentations than might be expected.

Freud's structural model pointed towards another way of looking at the ego's problems in psychosis. The ego arises, according to Freud's structural model, from the perceptual apparatus, or it grows out of that apparatus. Thus there is a fundamental problem for the ego when, in psychosis, it has to break with the reality that its perception presents. It has to accomplish a severe distortion, which alienates the ego from its origins in perception. This coming apart of the ego weakens it. In the 1930s the Viennese psychoanalysts emphasised the problem of the ego's 'synthetic function' (Rado 1928, Nunberg 1931): to be able to hold things together under tension, especially the tension between the id and the super-ego. To reconcile these two adequately is a mark of ego-strength. In the psychoses, the ego has a weakness in this respect.

In neurosis the ego is stronger. It can cope with its Oedipal conflicts, albeit with the use of repression. In schizophrenia, it is not merely a conflict that has to be dealt with, but a weakness in the ego (Wexler 1971). When a conflict increases above a certain intensity, the ego's synthetic function fails, and cannot resolve the conflict. Instead the ego is overwhelmed by the conflict and ultimately by unconscious, primary-process functioning. Consciously there is then a manifestation of primary-process thinking dominated by unruly displacements and condensations, and a lack of proper coherence.

In this view the boundary of repression is weaker in psychotic patients than in normal persons. Primary-process thought seems to emerge as if the psychotic has only a delicate membrane easily permeable to primary process, when conflicts and tensions rise. In those acute episodes the ego cannot adequately keep to the separation of unconscious from conscious.

This notion of a weak ego that is hard pressed to keep primary process at bay led to certain considerations of treatment. Classical technique needed to be modified. Federn (1934) warned of the particularly detrimental consequences of regression in psychosis, and how to prevent that by avoiding free associations and being openly self-revealing about the countertransference. Wexler (1965), on the grounds that the ego has a deficit, recommended a sort of ego training and support, like bringing up a child, using 'education, restriction of destructive impulses, support, affection, and the provision of effective models for thought, feeling, and action. Even the bolstering of the defensive organization' (Wexler 1965, p. 286). Eissler concluded that in the acute phase of schizophrenia, the patient does not respond to secondary-process functioning in his environment; so, the analyst has to use his own primary process, i.e. his intuition about the primary process in his environment. However, as Eissler cryptically says, 'The problem then is that of using the primary processes rationally, i.e. to the greatest possible benefit of the acutely sick patient '(Eissler 1951, p. 145). Somewhat similarly, Rosen (1947) described an approach he called direct analytic therapy, in which underlying instinctual drives are interpreted and discussed: a procedure frowned upon in the analysis of neurotics. Such modifications of technique have led to the criticism that these analysts are no longer conducting a psychoanalysis (Rosenfeld 1952).

Omnipotence and identity

The disorder that Segal identified as the problem behind symbol formation in schizophrenia was one of identity. There is no proper distinction between the symbol itself, the thing represented and the person using the symbol. Segal thought that the mechanisms involved in this had the quality of omnipotence. The symboliser equates the symbol with the thing symbolised on the basis that the symboliser identifies himself/herself with other persons. This kind of identification is characterised as omnipotent because the phantasy and attitudes involved can actually dissolve the boundaries between one person and another as if the thought has really achieved the effect (see Freud's case of the Ratman (Freud 1909b) for his original description of omnipotent thinking and omnipotent phantasies). Thus a schizophrenic may announce that he *is* Napoleon; just as one of Segal's (1957; see also 'Projective identification and symbolic relations', above) schizophrenic patients equated 'violin' with his own genitals. Such an omnipotent equation not only makes symbols very concrete, but also greatly distorts personal identity.

This kind of omnipotent identification was widely explored by Herbert Rosenfeld, who described 'omnipotent narcissistic object-relations' (Rosenfeld 1964). That kind of omnipotence takes the form of a projective intrusion into others with the aim of abolishing any separation that might provoke anxiety or envy.

> In narcissistic object relations defences against any recognition of separateness between self and object play a predominant part. Awareness of separation would lead to feelings of dependence on an object and therefore to anxiety . . . The omnipotent narcissistic object relations therefore obviate both the aggressive feelings caused by frustration and any awareness of envy. (Rosenfeld 1964, p. 333)

Because projective identification involves the attribution of a part of oneself to another, it allows a kind of belief that one actually *is* that other person in some respect (see also Klein's paper on identification, 1955). This points towards the obvious difficulties that schizophrenics have in establishing a real sense of identity.[4]

These distortions of identity brook no questioning and demand a recognition that the way things appear to that person is exactly and incontrovertibly so. That person will then proceed on the basis that it is so – and when such beliefs are entertained about himself, he behaves in a way that is just as he believes himself to be. Many theoretical views regard omnipotent belief systems as part of schizophrenia, from Freud's analysis of Schreber to schizophrenic symbol formation, to Winnicott's pinpointing of infantile omnipotence (towards which we will make our way below).

The existential problem

Problems with a sense of personal identity form another starting point to understand the experience of schizophrenia. Some theories of schizophrenia take the identity problem, rather than the thought disorder, as central. The schizophrenic suffers an existential sense of not being real, or not feeling properly in existence. For instance, it is not uncommon for schizophrenic patients to identify with Hamlet and his existential angst about being and not being.

A patient I encountered many years ago told me his identity was 'not-Hamlet', and he wanted his file changed to that effect. We can

4 There is a useful contrasting comparison to be made with empathy, which might be thought of as a *non-omnipotent* form of projective identification into someone else. With empathy I put myself in another's shoes. I can see someone else's predicament without losing sight of my own similar experience, or memory. Empathy is an active attempt to relate to another person's troubles or feelings while retaining a sense of my own feelings being mine; I retain a sense of having those feelings in my own life and life situations. It is possible, and in fact common, to connect with another person's bereavement by recalling a bereavement of one's own in the past. The contrast to be made with an omnipotent form of identification is experiencing another's grief in such a way that the experience of grief becomes distant and alien. Only the other person really *suffers* grief. Or, in another context, I can attribute guilt to another person for driving badly, while completely exonerating myself. In that case, any sense I might have of guilt vanishes in the process of attributing all guilt to the other motorist. On a wider stage, it is an irony that Hitler condemned Jews for a conspiracy to take over the world, while overlooking his own ambitions in that direction. The person escaping grief will behave as if he is no longer bereaved, or the bad car-driver behaves as if without faults; Hitler behaved as if his desire for world domination was not a guilty conspiracy, only that ascribed to the Jews.

see that he tried to explain that he was a Hamlet who had decided the question (to be or not to be) in favour of not-being. I believe now that he was saying he felt a non-person. However, at the time, in my perplexity, I could only see him as thought-disordered. Acquiescingly, he went along with that, thus demonstrating again his inability to stand up for his own experience – an experience of non-identity in this case.

The most powerful statement of this approach in psychiatry was made in 1960 by R.D. Laing, to celebrated acclaim. Laing's reference point is, explicitly, existential philosophy – Kierkegaard, Heidegger, Sartre – fashionable in the 1950s. He was briefly a psychoanalyst and his ideas bear the hallmarks of British object-relations psychoanalysis.

There is an intense humanism in this thinking, and an attempt to stay close to the schizophrenic's experience. The core idea in Laing's argument is that the schizophrenic patient, when interviewed by his psychiatrist, expresses in somewhat coded ways his experience, right now, of being with the psychiatrist. Often he protests, in disguised ways. Often the protest is against being interviewed in a standard psychiatric manner, and it is often mocking, as in the vivid material that Kraepelin (1905) reported and Laing reviewed. Kraepelin's description is thus:

> The patient I will show you today has almost to be carried into the room, as he walks in a straddling fashion on the outside of his feet. On coming in, he throws off his slippers, sings a hymn loudly, and then cries twice (in English), 'My father, real father!' He is eighteen years old, and a pupil of the Oberrealschule (higher-grade modern-side school), tall, and rather strongly built, but with a pale complexion, on which there is often a transient flush. The patient sits with his eyes shut, and pays no attention to his surroundings. He does not look up even when he is spoken to, but he answers beginning in a low voice, and gradually screaming louder and louder. When asked where he is, he says, 'You want to know that too? I tell you who is being measured and is measured and shall be measured. I know all that, and could tell you, but I do not want to.' When asked his name he screams, 'What is your name? What does he shut? He shuts his eyes. What does he hear? He does not understand; he understands not. How? Who? Where? When? What does he mean? When I tell him to look he does not look properly. You there,

> just look! What is it? What is the matter? Attend; he attends not. I say, what is it, then? Why do you give me no answer? Are you getting impudent again? How can you be so impudent? I'm coming! I'll show you! You don't whore for me. You mustn't be smart either; you're an impudent, lousy fellow, such an impudent lousy fellow I've never met with. Is he beginning again? You understand nothing at all, nothing at all; nothing at all does he understand. If you follow now, he won't follow, will not follow. Are you getting still more impudent? Are you getting impudent still more? How they attend, they do attend, and so on.' At the end he scolds in quite inarticulate sounds. (Kraepelin 1905, pp. 79–80; quoted in Laing 1960, pp. 29–30).

Kraepelin presented this as an example of the *non sequiturs* and incomprehensibility of the schizophrenic. So much for Kraepelin's account; Laing perceptively reinterpreted:

> The construction we put on this behaviour will, however, depend on the relationship we establish with the patient . . . Surely [the patient] is carrying on a dialogue between his own parodied version of Kraepelin, and his own defiant, rebellious self. (Laing 1960, p. 30)

Laing's interest is in the schizophrenic's experience of being a person within the whole field of study; and that whole field includes the encounter between the two parties, the psychiatrist and the patient. While the psychiatrist was observing the patient, his behaviour and the signs and symptoms of schizophrenia, the patient was studying the psychiatrist and the attempts, if any, to appreciate the schizophrenic's experience. Laing drew attention to the fact that one party to this observation (Kraepelin) is quite unaware that the other is also studying the situation. Laing stressed the psychiatrist's typical lack of awareness of the schizophrenic's sensitivity to his (the psychiatrist's) own behaviour. He documents the patient's despair, ridicule, rebellion and so on, which the complacent psychiatrist misinterpreted as psychopathology. Curiously, whereas the usual assumption in psychiatry is that the psychotic is cut off from his surroundings, Laing argued that the schizophrenic is hypersensitive and reactive to his own surroundings, in particular the psychiatrist himself. Laing owed a good deal to the psychoanalytic revolution of the 1950s, in which countertransference came to the fore (Heimann 1950; Racker 1968) and psychoanalysis became sensitised to the analyst as an active element in the psychoanalytic setting. While psychoanalysis may have moved more and more towards understanding this interaction of the unconscious of two subjects, psychiatry seems to have moved in the opposite direction: to greater neglect of the interpersonal encounter and an emphasis on objectifying the subject, the schizophrenic (e.g. Martinez-Hernaez 2000).

Laing proceeded from the clinical context, to conduct much more widespread research into the families of schizophrenics (Laing and Esterson 1964). He connected with the work being conducted at the time (in the 1950s and 1960s) by Ackerman (1958), Lidz (1963) and others. His work was also adjacent to the influential but non-psychoanalytic work of Bateson *et al.* (1956).

The double bind

Bateson defined the 'double bind' (Bateson *et al.* 1956). This is based on communication theory. The schizophrenic is believed to have suffered an identity problem in the course of her upbringing in a family that consistently operates conflicted messages *at different levels of abstraction* simultaneously through different channels of communication.

Bateson started with the idea of the 'category mistake' as described by Russell (Whitehead and Russell 1910), which stated that a category of things cannot itself be a member of that category. The category of even numbers cannot itself be a member of that category; so, the category of even numbers cannot be an even number. Applied to communication in schizophrenic families, Bateson believed that an explicit verbal communication (say, a mother telling her son off) carried non-verbal clues that stated another message at another level of abstraction (say, mothers never get angry with their sons). If he is specifically given to understand he is a bad boy, while another more abstract communication insists that mothers never think their sons are bad, then he cannot locate himself consistently within the experiential world of his family. He loses a purchase on the nature of his own identity and being. Thus, the son is not just put into a conflict, but is confused over the nature of his own experiences and his identity, reflected back to him quite differently in different levels of communication. There is a specific level and an abstract level of communications. This son angers his mother, but sons never anger their mothers; therefore what sort of son is he? Bateson concluded that this cognitive dissonance over the person's very identity was the key to the schizophrenic's identity problem. This notion of the double bind has often been degraded to mean simple conflicts, but it refers explicitly to the confusion of levels of abstraction to which the child is subjected in his family about his existence and identity. The result is that the child also lacks the capacity to master abstract thought properly. The concrete thinking typical of a schizophrenic arises from a taught confusion about levels of abstraction. He is subjected to a confusion about how to describe his world, and how to experience himself in his reactions to the world of his family. This theory has the benefit of probing the existential sense of being in the world, as well as the cognitive deficit.

The mirror stage

Bateson, like Laing, was influential in 1950s and 1960s psychiatry. There is a similarity also with the views of Lacan on the mirror stage in development (Lacan 1949) in which the infant, having some sense of himself, begins to recognise an external, objective image of himself, as in a mirror. His parents, as if a mirror, donate to his identity all sorts of properties defined by society that the infant does not appreciate through his own experience of himself subjectively. The social imposition is characteristically mediated through language and the implicit assumptions about human being and doing that are conveyed in the structure of a language. Lacan stressed the strong linguistic or semiotic structure.

The infant begins to know himself (i.e. reflect on himself) and his instinctual impulses through the defining mirror of language. The mirror is a kind of interlocutor, which Lacan said has an aspect of prohibition and boundary-keeping. That prohibitive element is a kind of father who threatens castration as punishment for transgressions. In particular, the father is responsible for insisting on language and its rules. The individual enters on his social future through language and is impelled into it through the rule of the father. This is argued, by Lacan, to be a general paradox for all human development; the paradox of the infant's awareness of himself subjectively, and his awareness through the social mirror of father's language. Therefore, it does not carry the specificity that would be required to explain the occurrence of schizophrenia in only some of the general population. Schizophrenia must result instead from a more primary problem. That problem is concerned with the origins of the mirror phase.

Specifically, psychosis results from the obliteration of this father from the experience of a child – Lacan used a term of Freud's which he translated as *forclosion* in French ('foreclosure'), the cancelling or elimination of the father and particularly of the possibility of castration. As a result a hole appears at the centre of the person's developing being, and a distortion of language develops (Lacan 1955–1956).

Lacan's views on the mirror stage were known to Winnicott when he also described the role of mirroring in the development of the infant (Winnicott 1967). Winnicott described the mother's gaze as a mirror for the child. Mother's reactions in whatever mode – visual, auditory or tactile – give signals to the infant of its own state and its existence. A depressed mother is likely, through her numbed responses, to convey deadness to the infant, or maybe non-existence. For Winnicott, the mother is required to replay to the infant certain important characteristics of the infant. First of all, at the outset of the life of the infant, she must confirm the infant's sense of its own omnipotence. He described the infant as starting life with an illusory omnipotence, and each infant *needs* to sustain that delusion for a certain period. If for instance the very young infant feels hungry then it is important for the mother to offer a feed – say, the breast – in such a way that the infant can feel it conjured up the breast for itself in order to supply its own hunger. Mother must do nothing to interrupt that innate illusion, or 'primary omnipotence' as Winnicott called it; 'when things go well the infant has no means of knowing what is being properly provided' (Winnicott 1960, p. 52). Subsequently, mother has the task of introducing the infant, by graduated steps, to the reality of its actual helplessness. This is no mean task for a mother. Gradually mother must fail to support the illusion – for instance by leaving the baby to wait before it is fed. The mother's role is then to be only an imperfect mother – a 'good-enough mother' and this supplies the infant with graduated doses of its own helplessness, from which the infant can then gradually appreciate the enormity of reality. However, for infants who go on to become psychotic, this process goes badly wrong. The mirror is not a gentle lead towards the reality of dependence.

Impingement

Winnicott (1960) then postulated a mother who does not fail in this graduated way, but allows a major failure. Her failure is more than the minimal graduations of a good-enough mother. Mother's failure, he said, does not cause an appreciation of reality. Instead it results in a traumatic rent in the illusion of the omnipotent self. Winnicott called this an 'impingement' of the environment upon the fragile infantile sense of self. He said that it causes a break in the 'continuity of being'. That 'central core of the ego is affected, and this is the very nature of psychotic anxiety' (Winnicott 1960, pp. 46–47). He was here describing the existential disaster of the schizophrenic: 'Anxiety in these early stages . . . relates to the threat of annihilation' (Winnicott 1960, p. 47). He explicitly related this break in the continuity of being to the development of schizophrenia. Thereafter the developing infant, child, and later the adult, have a serious defect in, or complete absence of, an identity. They can only cover over this break by some kind of false sense of self. Typically, the false self is an attempt to fit into some part that others want, a social role. That sense of being comes from others, from outside. A social role stands in for a personal identity. The inner central core of a self is lost. People who lack that inner sense of self are therefore extremely fragile and extremely dependent on others. Winnicott comes very close to Freud's understanding of Schreber's attempts to recreate a world, in describing recovery as the creation of a false self. However, in Winnicott's case, the false self is an adaptation to external demands of others. The elusive (prematurely destroyed) feeling of omnipotence is pursued through the notion that one's identity consists precisely in giving others what they demand. The person is then very vulnerable, since the loss of the external support to his identity, a failure to *be* that identity for others, threatens annihilation of omnipotence and of the self, and the onset of psychosis.

Often the notion of a false self is used as if it were to conceal a true self, but that would be more like the persona of a neurotic who represses his own authenticity in some respect. In Winnicott's theory of psychosis the false self is applied to cover over a gap, a place where there is *no* true self. This contrasts with the 'gap' or 'lack' that Lacan specified, where the infant lacks a proper defining environment such that the absence of a linguistic 'law of the father' denies the infant the framework to know his personal identity.

Interestingly, all these attempts to approach the existential collapse of the schizophrenic, although sometimes contradictory, locate the origins of schizophrenia in interpersonal causes. Attractive though this may be in some respects, it is not attractive to the mothers or families of schizophrenics, who feel overly responsible for this interpersonal causation of psychosis. Nor does it accord with psychiatric research into the genetic and biological factors in schizophrenia. Of course, the role of genetic and physical factors has been curiously elusive; so elusive to modern scientific methods over such a long period that it raises suspicions that there is no physical basis. Actually, epidemiological studies of families, and twins, infer some innate, internal determining factor. Acceptance of an innate factor suggests some innate psychoanalytic equivalent, for which death instinct (a Kleinian view) or an inherent ego-weakness (an ego-psychology view) are the best candidates. Because of the emphasis by many psychoanalytic authors that the interpersonal dimension is determinant, biologically oriented psychiatrists have viewed psychoanalysis with increasing suspicion. This cleavage between biological and psychodynamic psychiatry has been particularly noticeable in the USA, because psychoanalysis was at one time (1950s to 1970s) so influential in psychiatry there. Now the two sides of psychiatry are diverging rapidly, as in many other countries (see 'Schisms' in Essay 3, p. 119, for an extended discussion of this schismatic process).

Interpersonal relations

A dominant trend in American psychoanalysis in the 1930s developed a particularly strong interpersonal emphasis. This prompted Freda Fromm-Reichman (1939) to reconsider psychoanalytic technique with schizophrenics. She recommended that interpretation should no longer be the key to therapy, the analyst's emotional sensitivity being more important:

> the schizophrenic patient and the therapist are people living in different worlds and on different levels of personal development with different means of expressing and of orienting themselves. We know little about the language of the unconscious of the schizophrenic, and our access to it is blocked by the very process of our own adjustment to a world the schizophrenic has relinquished. So we should not be surprised that errors and misunderstandings occur when we undertake to communicate and strive for a rapport with him. (Fromm-Reichman 1939, p. 416)

The world view of the psychotic is extraordinarily remote from that of the psychoanalyst or psychiatrist. The analyst's responsibility is to enter the patient's world with complete accuracy. The analyst must recognise the stretch of imagination necessary, and the extreme sensitivity of the schizophrenic to one's mistakes and incomprehension.

The schizophrenic patient is particularly unreliable in his reactions, and expresses himself in terms of symbolic gestures or sounds that take the analyst who is used to the neurotic by surprise. 'The technique we use with psychotics is different from our approach to psychoneurotics. This is . . . due to his extremely intense and sensitive transference reactions' (Fromm-Reichman 1939, p. 412). The psychotic has an extremely fragile 'self' which must be protected and conserved at all costs. Thus, Fromm-Reichman attributes problems in therapy to mistakes in the analyst's understanding. This corresponds closely to Laing's account of Kraepelin's case (see above).

This tradition looked to Harry Stack Sullivan (Sullivan 1962). Sullivan worked with Fromm-Reichman at Chestnut Lodge, the in-patient clinic established to treat schizophrenic patients psychoanalytically. He inspired a following with his theories of interpersonal relations and, like American psychoanalysis in general before the Second World War, he was independent, unconventional and pragmatic. Sullivan's practice, based on interpersonal awareness, was exemplified in Fromm-Reichman's approach above. He recommended this interpersonal sensitivity as a need to attend to the patient's 'self-system' *within* the setting of the psychoanalytic interview. Sullivan's interpersonal approach downplayed the intrapsychic dimension, so that he saw the schizophrenic disturbance in terms of the patient's social relations, which implicated group, social and cultural issues extensively. Sullivan's inspirational influence on American psychoanalysis was eventually overshadowed in the 1940s by the *émigré* European analysts, who set out to eradicate indigenous American psychoanalysis.

However, Sullivan's influence endured in the later development of self-psychology and the currently fashionable interpersonal school (Levenson 1992), and the intersubjective school (Atwood and Stolorow 1984, Renik 1993). Harold Searles, interested in the interpersonal quality of the psychoanalytic setting, led a way back to a more rigorous understanding of the intra-psychic aspects (Searles 1979). Willing to confide his own countertransference reactions to the patient, Searles saw his job as enabling the patient to 'come increasingly to exchange his erstwhile autistic world for the world consisting of, and personified by, the analyst' (Searles 1979, p. 190). These authors seek in one way, more or less psychoanalytically, to reintroduce the patient to a world inhabited by other persons, or at least the world of the one other person the patient is acquainted with in psychoanalysis, i.e. the analyst. They directly address a radical disjunction that was so trenchantly demarcated by Laing, the disjunction between the patient's view of the psychiatrist and the psychiatrist's view of the patient. That disjunction, they claim, is the instigator of symptoms. The analyst must almost fall over backwards to accommodate the patient, and to connect him in a kind of birth ceremony back to the analyst's world. In all this, as Fromm-Reichman proposed, there is a tendency to abandon the unconscious and to resort to active techniques to overcome the disjunction of worlds.

Interpersonal approaches take their starting point in the technical difficulties of relating to schizophrenics – or rather the patients' difficulties in relating with the analyst. They challenge Freud's view that the patient does not relate. Instead these psychoanalysts start with the view that the schizophrenic does in fact relate, and does so very intensely. The problem is on the other side – it is the problem of the analyst to relate to the patient with the degree of sensitivity necessary to make the patient feel understood. The starting point is the same as Freud's – the relatedness problem – but the approach is to achieve, in a direct way, the missing relationship, and to understand how it is embedded in the subtle though bizarre behaviour of the schizophrenic. This solution entails an engaging humility – the problem becomes the analyst's. That is to say, the analyst must break through the relationship impasse as a technical procedure. Her job is not to construct a metapsychological understanding of the schizophrenic mind, but to construct a sort of halfway world in which the schizophrenic can begin to resume human relations. In the end, we might wonder how much the wish to create this world of extremely careful attention focused on the schizophrenic entails a kind of collusive partnership based on the schizophrenic's narcissistic wish for a recreated world to his liking.

The findings are quite the opposite of Freud's – the schizophrenic does indeed relate, often tenaciously, to the analyst, and with a great and destabilising sensitivity. The necessary modification of technique has been criticised as abandoning the psychoanalytic method:

> Most American psycho-analytical workers on schizophrenia, for example, Harry Stack Sullivan, Fromm-Reichmann, Federn, Knight, Wexler, Eissler, and Rosen, etc., have changed their method of approach so considerably that it can no longer be called psycho-analysis. They seem all agreed that it is futile to regard the psycho-analytical method as useful for acute psychosis. They all find re-education and reassurance absolutely necessary; some workers like Federn go so far as to think that the positive transference has to be fostered and the negative one avoided altogether. He also warns us against interpreting unconscious material. (Rosenfeld 1952, p. 111)

In terms of psychosis, American pragmatism – doing what works – seems in practice to have affected the purist *émigré* Europeans. Before the 1940s, the boundaries between psychoanalysis and psychotherapy were much less distinct, and parameters such as the use of the couch, non-interpretative interventions and personal confidences were much more relaxed with psychotic patients. The emphasis was pragmatic. Despite their purism, the incoming Viennese ego-psychologists did, themselves, recommend pragmatic changes, as we saw in 'Synthetic function and ego weakness' (p. 70).

All these authors in America addressed less directly the specific cognitive deficit, the strange symbolisations and the existential gap, since they concentrated on establishing a relationship and sustaining it. Nevertheless, there are theoretical assumptions behind these innovations in technique. Sullivan replaced Freud's metapsychology with his own. He abandoned a commitment to the sexual libido as the fundamental drive in human nature – or at least the one most susceptible to causing pathology – and replaced it with a basic drive towards growth and maturation.

> When we come to Sullivan's theory of personality, however, we find a definite deviation from Freud's thinking . . . The basic difference is in a different philosophy of personality development . . . Sullivan also starts with the assumption of a basic drive in man – one towards growth and maturation . . . Sexual maturation would be but one aspect of this drive. Having postulated this basic need for growth, his interest then shifts to a study of the acculturation process . . . So while Freud sees the child's development as going on inevitably in terms of the child's sexual development and his libido, Sullivan's child is a product of his

> interaction with significant people. He assumes that the need for security is even stronger in the human being than the need for instinctual gratification or satisfaction and that these latter become problems only when they conflict with the need for security . . . [A]ccording to Sullivan [we must] concern ourselves chiefly with the forces which do dominate man, and they are the social forces. (Thompson 1978, pp. 494–495)

Sullivan's approach was essentially social, though he retained the psychoanalytic notation of the unconscious, repression and transference.

This completes my review of the most significant attempts to understand the schizophrenic experience. Certain issues about the nature of clinical understanding remain to be mentioned before we turn to an extended illustration of some of the theoretical points we have covered.

Understanding as a defence

Sullivan's injunction was to understand as a strategy of relating, rather than as a strategy for knowledge and insight. His approach, and schizophrenia in general, raises issues about the nature, and especially the purpose, of understanding. Understanding may simply be gratifying; for example, Steiner (1993) makes

> a distinction between *understanding* and *being understood* . . . the patient who is not interested in acquiring understanding – that is, in understanding himself – may yet have a pressing need to be understood. (Steiner 1993, p. 132)

The analyst gratifies the patient by agreeing to *be* his self-understanding, instead of that knowledge being owned by the patient. The alternative approach is to understand what has happened to the patient's own self-understanding, and why. So, we need a certain circumspection and caution about entering the world of the psychotic. For what purpose do we try to understand him? Because of the intolerable pain, the psychotic has blown his mind in order to avoid knowing himself. The analyst might also take due care in approaching that pain. So, there may be not merely difference of meaning, but also different worlds of assumptions and experiences between analyst and patient about the need to understand. The patient may agree to being understood so long as he does not have to do the understanding. In Essay 1, we saw how psychiatric staff have to be their patient's self-knowledge, and self-care, and Conran described how uncomfortable that could be (see 'Who knows?', p. 18). Psychoanalysts, too, may be defensive – in their own way. For instance, one evasion might be the distortion of understanding that comes from focusing on the meaning of a patient's symptoms, rather than finding meaning in her experiences and relationships. In that case there is an easy kind of meaning.[5] Consider the following vignette:

> A patient on admission angrily said, 'I am God's older brother'. I replied that he must really be fed up with his younger brother getting all the publicity! The patient stopped, smiled and a mutual warmth developed between us from that time onwards. Previously he had taken his brother's car and driven it into a wall, fortunately without any resulting injury. He thought he was omnipotent; that at the time, he could do anything. (Lucas 2003, p. 5)

The analyst's joke is a good one and funny. It amused the patient and, apparently, led to an enduring warm relationship between patient and analyst. This is a good rapport. However, the rapport is not on the basis of the patient's omnipotent murderousness towards his brother, which initially we must assume was so dreadful that the patient preferred to go mad. Both analyst and patient in this vignette preferred to enjoy a meaningful joke, and thus to distance themselves from the dreadful and omnipotent side of the patient. As Lucas explains: 'we always need to think in terms of two separate parts, the psychotic and the non-psychotic, not one person' (p. 5); and he would I think agree that his rapport with his patient was with the non-psychotic part of the person. In terms of the present argument, the choice of which part of the patient to link with is influenced strongly by a wish on the part of both not to engage too deeply with the psychotic terror, omnipotence and destruction. It reflects some

5 In Essay 1 we dissected out the three forms of meaning (see 'Action in understanding', p. 22): diagnostic meaning, reflective understanding of experience, and a kind of non-symbolic communication of meaning in actions. Here is a fourth variant, in which a kind of meaning is generated that is easy, and designed to keep distance from a much more painful meaning. It is a defensive meaning.

kind of resort to avoidance of pain, and it would seem that a psychoanalyst is no less tempted than any other psychiatric carer.

To receive real conscious meaning about his suffering would surely lead the patient to a good deal of suffering.

> While on the ward, for months, [a young woman] kept denying any problems. One weekend, she went home to her mother and jumped out of her bedroom window, fracturing her leg. While still on the orthopaedic ward she came to see me in my out-patient clinic. She was in a frightened state and asked to be readmitted to the mental hospital, on medical discharge.
>
> When she returned to the mental hospital, she reverted to a denial of any problems. Anti-psychotic medication was having no effect on her mental state. I then realised that she hadn't jumped out of the window in a state of despair, she had been pushed out by an intolerant [psychotic] part.
>
> When I put this to her, her mental state suddenly changed. She made out that she was religious and that I was a bigot and intolerant of religion. (Lucas 2003, p. 6)

Quite clearly the analyst did eventually touch in some way the psychotic part of the patient, which reacted accordingly. There was no warm rapport this time. The patient's real difficulty with psychic truth came out in a quite different way from the easy interpretation of Lucas' previous vignette.

In this sense, the psychoanalyst can be tempted to pursue the meanings of symptoms rather than the meaning of the pain of the patient. It is only too understandable. For the first of Lucas' patients, the meaning of the symptom (the patient's delusional identity) circumvented the point of pain for the patient. Taking such a distance from the pain of psychosis, which that patient invited, compares with general psychiatrists giving meaning in the form of a diagnostic label. The psychiatrist and his patient are also occupied with finding meaning, but the psychiatrist finds meaning in generalisation, for instance the constellations of symptoms that *mean* a diagnosis. Distance from the existential suffering is created by seeking the generalities of professional diagnosis. The defensive use of psychoanalytic meanings is not generalising, and remains particular for a patient; however, both strategies can feel meaningful and reassuring, and comfort both patient and carer. In contrast, engaging with the psychotic part of the patient touches on pain, and results in a seriously disconcerting effect that disturbs both. Such a contrasting meaning occurred with Lucas' second patient.

Hermeneutics

A rather different frame of reference – hermeneutics – is relevant here. I have pursued the question as to whether understanding and meaning can be easy and used to avoid pain, or, contrastingly, to approach the pain that is avoided. There may be a comforting virtue in the former, if the pain is too great. However, the hermeneutic frame of reference would hold that there is no 'true' pain in the sense that I am implying. The need the psychoanalyst supplies is simply to find meaning itself. Absence of meaning is the pathology. The pathology can be righted simply by supplying a meaningful narrative of a person's life. In this sense meanings would always be a relief. This view of psychoanalysis (see Riccoeur 1981; Habermas 1971) does have a benign charm, as it seems to obviate hidden suffering, or the pain of disclosing trauma and anxiety. Psychoanalysis would then be something like supplying vitamins to someone who is vitamin-deficient – it gives meaning to the meaning-deficient. If that hermeneutic view of psychoanalysis were true, then the two vignettes of Lucas would not really be distinguishable. In fact, there is much psychoanalytic evidence to suggest that the meaning that psychoanalysis is concerned with is painful, and especially in work with psychotic patients. Moreover, easy meanings are probably defensive understanding, rather than supplying a psychic vitamin. Some evidence of this kind is apparent in the illustration that will follow in a moment.

Hence, psychoanalytic meaning in schizophrenia may be considered along several lines of thought. First, in the conventional psychoanalytic tradition, some authentic truth about the patient is destroyed as a defensive decathexis of reality (and then narcissistically reconstructed). Second, meaning is created as a collusive pseudo-understanding which avoids pain for both parties. Third, in the hermeneutic view, meaning of any kind is a psychic restorative which psychoanalysis can supply, but which has a looser connection with 'truth'.

Reflecting on the theories

I shall now take a published case of a young male schizophrenic, and discuss the account as it is given by Murray Jackson (Jackson and

Williams 1994, Chapter 2). I do so in order to illustrate some of the dimensions I have isolated from this theoretical account (see 'Dimensions of understanding', p. 49). The material lends itself to considering a number of these dimensions: interpersonal versus intra-psychic; existential suffering versus professional diagnosis; symbolism versus meaninglessness; misunderstandings versus self-destructiveness; interpreting meaning versus interpreting ego damage; the non-psychotic versus the psychotic parts of the self.

A case of schizophrenic self-burning

Anthony was 28, and had been a schizophrenic for 10 years following the death of his brother (older by 11 months) in a car accident. Anthony believed that God had left the world because of its greedy destructiveness, but he could save the world for God by burning himself to death. He had persistent self-burning impulses, and had made an attempt by pouring petrol on a hut which he set on fire with himself inside. He had been rescued but suffered severe burns.

On the ward, which Jackson ran as a psychodynamic assessment unit for young schizophrenics, the staff found the patient frightening: a menace that was sometimes expressed in a mock strangling of a nurse. Attempts to talk to him about his desperate feelings found him lofty in manner, full of mystic philosophising, and dismissive of enquiries. He believed that his feelings were located in his left leg.

Interpersonal or intra-psychic

The psychodynamic culture of the unit placed a lot of weight on a patient's account of his feelings. The assessment occupied two exploratory interviews conducted by Jackson. Early in the first interview, Anthony demonstrates his talent for rather superior mockery; for instance:

Anthony: I don't know what my emotions are like. I'm not in touch with my emotions. I think my ego has something to do with it. If I have an emotion, I get egotistical about it. I don't have emotions often. When I'm in a situation where I am aware of my emotions, I get egotistical buzzes. I'm pleased at having emotions. I think 'God. I'm great. I've had an emotion.' It's just a pleasure buzz, but it destroys

> the emotion, because the buzz becomes more important than the emotion. (Jackson and Williams 1994, p. 51)

Anthony is here conforming, in a way, to the rhetoric of feelings, or emotions, that occupies the ward culture. He is also conveying how he is emotionally distant from (maybe superior to) the emphasis on emotions. He conveys with some mockery how excited he is when he can produce an emotion as required. He says, as it were, that the triumph in doing what is required obliterates the feeling he is supposed to be expressing. This kind of mocking humour is similar to Kraepelin's patient, as revealed by Laing, in the quote earlier (see 'The existential problem', p. 73). Anthony leads his interviewer on:

Anthony: . . . I think my emotions are very mature and powerful now.
MJ: Mature and powerful? But not available to you. (p. 52)

Jackson is expressing a fundamental assumption of the unit culture – that feelings are so painful that they are rendered into some unavailable state.

Anthony: They're not available to me, no.
MJ: Where are they then to be found?
Anthony: They're about there *(points to about three feet to his left, in mid-air)*. When I feel an emotion, I bring it in from about there, and then into my body. My emotions are just there. There's a space which is isolated . . . my emotions are isolated from me by an intellectual barricade. It's just there. (p. 52)

Anthony is putting into very graphic and concrete terms a view based on that which he finds in the unit – feelings are isolated, and intellect can effect that distance, as if it were an effective defence (barricade) in Anthony's terms. Again, it is not obvious how much this is a mockery of the rather concrete way MJ thinks about an actual location where the feelings might be found. Then, after some animated interchanges between Anthony and the interviewer about his left leg and his emotions:

Anthony: . . . My left leg eludes analysis and always will, unless you chop it off and throw it away. I realise the futility of analysis. (p. 53)

And later, with some more exasperated irony:

Anthony: . . . We haven't talked about my emotional hang-ups, which is what I want to talk about. We've talked about shaking legs and my left leg. What am I to make of that? I'm here for healing, not in-depth analysis of my left leg.
MJ: Well, let's turn to your emotional hang-ups.
Anthony: Not unless you want to. If there's something else you'd rather like to talk about, please talk about it. (p. 54)

The interviewer acknowledges his own steering of the conversation towards the spatial representation of his feelings rather than their content; Anthony responds with a parody of a psychotherapist.

In these excerpts, we can see Anthony responding to the psychodynamic and cultural demands of the unit. These demand that he explore the internal relations the patient has with his feelings, and, with support, that he express them. Anthony continued after the interviewer's invitation, cited above, to talk of his delight in having fun with people, though most can't take it. He describes it as sounding like being a baby. The interviewer misses the possibility that Anthony may be talking of the fun he is having with the interviewer, and perseveres with great seriousness,

MJ: . . . When you said you felt like a baby, I'm not sure what sort of experience that is.
Anthony: I wanted to have fun, and it was a selfish thing to want. I felt isolated. I had no-one to have fun with.
MJ: Do you think that is something you also missed out in earlier life?
(Pause)
Anthony: Yes. That sounds true. (pp. 54–55)

There is a kind of tension here: the interviewer places the emphasis on the internal world of feelings and relations to them, and picks up on the idea that there is a 'baby' part of the patient that he needs to become acquainted with. The interviewer is following standard procedure for a psychodynamic assessment, and does it with astuteness. The tension arises in Anthony's playing with him, having fun at the interviewer's expense – and the interviewer seems to respond with a worthy seriousness, as if he can coax Anthony into a serious psychodynamically-inspired discussion.

The concern must be that, given Anthony's psychotic condition, the standard psychodynamic approach misses the mark. It appears at first sight to be just the kind of dissonance between the patient's experience and the professional's intentions that Laing described in Kraepelin's work, or Sullivan and Fromm-Reichman were drawing attention to. The patient responds directly to the external world in which he finds himself, right *now*, with the psychoanalyst.

In Kraepelin's case, the patient was diagnosed as irrational and psychotic when he was trying to express a parody of the psychiatrist. In the case we are now discussing, while not aiming at a diagnosis, the interviewer is thinking of a psychodynamic model of repressed emotions. However, the dissonance between patient and analyst is similar. When Anthony bluntly states that the interviewer is analysing his left leg, and not talking of what he, Anthony, wants to talk of, it exactly resembles the dilemma that Kraepelin's patient had with his psychiatrist. It is the conflict of approaches between the *intra-psychic* condition of the patient, as perceived by the professional, on one hand, and on the other, the schizophrenic's hopelessness in his wish to relate *interpersonally* to the person he is with, about his suffering. The patient's dilemma here is covered by humour of a quite ironic, mocking kind. Lucas' vignette quoted above (regarding 'God's older brother', p. 85) is unusual in that he found a way of sharing a joke with his schizophrenic patient. Usually the patient does a good job of the cover, and it leaves the interviewer on a different tack, without realising it. (The schizophrenic's use of humour, especially mockery, is not often appreciated – largely, I believe, because for the professional the patient's life-situation is so grave, it is no joke. Moreover, the patient gives no clues, such as smiling or laughing, though giggling is often reported, albeit solemnly designated as inappropriate affect.)

So there is a discrepancy between the two parties, a radical disjunction between patient and professional that Laing described as the core of the existential dilemma for the schizophrenic. The professional has his own ideas about schizophrenic suffering as a profound intra-psychic damage, while the patient wants some sense of understanding of his own experience. It seems to be compounded by the schizophrenic's inability to express himself directly, and by the fact that he is occupied only by the immediate sense of dissonance.

Existential suffering or professional diagnosis

In this case, the interviewer continues to grapple with an interview that is going wrong, and does come closer to the patient. At the point we left them, the interviewer was hunting around for some handle of understanding. So, going back to that point:

MJ: . . . When you said you felt like a baby, I'm not sure what sort of experience that is.
Anthony: I wanted to have fun, and it was a selfish thing to want. I felt isolated. I had no-one to have fun with.
MJ: Do you think that is something you also missed out in earlier life?
(Pause)
Anthony: Yes. That sounds true.
MJ: That sounds true. Why was it the case?
Anthony: I don't know. I've never thought about it before. *(Pause)* I know I was silent for the first two years of life.
MJ: Silent?
Anthony: I didn't talk or do anything. My mother told me. I didn't say anything till I was two. I have some memories, but you know there's no real fun there. Things weren't right. (p. 55)

Here the interviewer is trying to follow Anthony by picking up on a sense of something missed out in his life. Anthony describes two years that were 'missing', as it were, at the beginning of his life. Clearly, it touched something in Anthony. He moved the discussion on a bit. It is as if Anthony is trying more seriously to engage the interviewer. It remains rather on the interviewer's terms, because the psychoanalyst is thinking about the early environment: was Anthony's mother somehow out of touch with her baby? This is close enough to the patient's immediate feeling right now that there is an analyst (substituting for mother) who has somehow been out of touch with his patient. So, Anthony can at least feel that the analyst may be able to put words to the problem, whether it is located now or then. Anthony expresses his inarticulateness; he can't talk of the problem directly – he couldn't as a baby, and probably can't now.

To the credit of the psychoanalyst, he is trying to move towards the patient's experience, though at this stage it is still in his own terms; terms that refer to early problems in mothering and maternal understanding. Also, Anthony is not expressing things quite in his own way. He is using his mother's reported memory. Perhaps this indicates his inability to grasp things for himself; he can only know himself through what he is told, a kind of mirror function that he needs interpersonally. Extrapolating a bit, it could go on to indicate his diminished sense of self; the loss of, or break in, his 'continuity of being', as Winnicott put it. That lack of continuity is expressed as a silence, as Anthony puts it. In addition, the question remains as to whether the 'memory' of his mother's memory is a reference to Anthony's experience now. It is called a memory because it is essentially a rather distanced piece of experience; it can be conjectured or imagined but the 'feelings' are silenced.

One of the theoretical questions is whether we are dealing with a conflict or a deficit. Do we have to reach and address the contents of the ego, or a deficit in the ego? Is it something amiss with the structure or function of the ego itself that makes conflict-resolution impossible, or even irrelevant?

Anthony's silence corresponds in some respects to Freud's 'first phase' of psychosis in which some essential thing is missing. The world, in Schreber's case, had been destroyed. This missing place in Anthony's experience cannot, by definition, be articulated. It leaves the analyst to pick his own way forward, and naturally he does so with his own psychoanalytic approach. Anthony's problem here is how to convey something to the interviewer, when Anthony cannot grasp what it is he needs to convey. He has tried to 'help' with mockery when things go wrong. And now he indicates a silence, a wordlessness, which Lacan might designate as 'foreclosure'. The problem for the analyst is whether to fill this gap with his own anticipated knowledge. The alternative to the psychoanalyst's knowledge is to 'stay with' the meaninglessness of the silence that cannot be given words.

Symbolism or meaninglessness

Following Anthony's last comment, the interviewer continues to build up a picture of Anthony's experience. The sense is that he is somewhat at a loss, and he casts about for significant questions to keep Anthony reflecting on his life experience:

Anthony: I didn't talk or do anything. My mother told me. I didn't say anything till I was two. I have some memories, but you know there's no real fun there. Things weren't right.

MJ: What's your memory of when things seemed to be alright last?

(Pause)

Anthony: I don't know. A long time ago. *(Pause)* I don't think things have ever been right.

(Pause)

MJ: That raises the question of what effect you think your brother's death had on you. What do you think about that? (p. 55)

The interviewer is still interested in the 'things' that weren't right. He takes a leap to Anthony's brother's death, as if immediately to supply something that *could* be put into words. The brother's death in a car accident was surely something that was 'not right'. When Anthony had said that things were never right, he seemed to be referring to the preceding remarks about not speaking. Thus we could consider that Anthony is still trying to convey something that could never be put into words, something that was not right in him or in his life. However, the interviewer's hunch about the brother suggests the view that the thing that is not right *could* be put into words.

This demonstrates two different possible versions of schizophrenia. One version, the interviewer's, is that hidden meanings exist in neurosis or dreams as symbols that represent repressed material in the unconscious. In this case, the brother's death is the silent thing not spoken about in the family, and repressed in Anthony. It was this view – that unconscious meanings exist to be interpreted – that brought Jung enthusiastically to Freud. It continues in some contemporary approaches to psychosis, such as those of some ego-psychologists. The second version is that something is essentially lost, has no meaning. Meaning has gone. It is not repressed. A gap remains, a silence, a lack of words. Then to supply a meaning is a comforting reassurance (for both parties), but it is not an interpretation. It is more of a sticking- plaster. If meaning is used as a sticking-plaster, it could give just the kind of assistance that an analyst gives to promote the second of Freud's stages, recreating a fill-in world.

What the interviewer is doing can then be looked at in either of two ways.

1 It is pointing to the hidden meaning – the trauma of Anthony's brother's death, the emotions connected to which have been

largely repressed. This corresponds to the attempts that some ego-psychologists make to give new strength to the ego, by encouraging the patient to find meaning. They function as an auxiliary ego that has more synthetic function than the patient.

2 It is an attempt to supply a meaning, to make up for Anthony, who has lost the capacity to generate a meaningful sense of himself. The interviewer in this second version is taking on himself the capacity for making meaning, and doing it *for* Anthony.

The second of these understandings of the interaction fits with Freud's account of the Schreber case, where the patient needed to reconstruct meaning to cover a gap in his ego function that has to be filled in with something meaningful. It could be likened to a sticking-plaster to cover a rent in the ego, that particular rent being the ego's loss of capacity to represent and symbolise for himself what has happened. What Freud showed was that Schreber reconstructed a world after it had suffered a catastrophe. It is therefore possible that the interviewer was in fact assisting this psychotic 'recovery' process, by offering a meaningful narrative that Anthony could not construct on his own, and indeed a reconstruction less idiosyncratic or alien to others.

The hermeneutic view of psychoanalysis (Riccoeur 1981; Habermas 1971) is that making meaning is exactly what the psychoanalytic method is. It holds that humans live by narrative, and we need to have a coherent one of ourselves and our lives. Patients in general, the hermeneuticist says, have lost meaningful narrative, and lost coherence in their lives and selves. Taken literally, this suggests that meaning itself is what the patient is after, and any meaning might do. On this basis, we could say that it is helpful for the schizophrenic patient to be supplied with meaning. The hermeneutic view is that it doesn't really matter whose meaning it is, if meaning itself is a cure. However, we have seen that it does seem to matter. Since the patient's meaning does not exist, it is inevitably the analyst's that will dominate, and if the analyst is patently dominant, this leads ultimately to mockery. Even if there is a sense of relief or reassurance for both parties when they have some coherent meaning – whether a psychoanalytic narrative or a psychiatrist's scientific diagnosis – there is still a patient who mocks the psychiatrist or analyst.

This argues against the view that any meaning is as good as any other. There was something the patient wanted to communicate. We can look at the progress of the interview after the psychoanalyst has supplied the brother's death as a possible meaningful event that touches on the core of silence. Anthony responds to the interviewer's suggestive pointing as follows:

MJ: That raises the question of what effect you think your brother's death had on you. What do you think about that?

Anthony: I don't know. I get egotistical buzzes about not feeling grief about him. That's why I don't enter into relationships, or have feelings. I didn't want buzzes about affection or humour or love. I wanted to have them straight. I don't want to start getting pleasure out of grief. (p. 55)

Anthony is back to his 'buzzes'. His response goes right back to the beginning of the interview. The talk about buzzes rather than feelings suggests a protest that he is not listened to and is inclined to mock again. Certainly Anthony is making a point about some sort of 'real' feelings that are missing, or silent, while his buzzes look like the mockery. The interview process must have reverted to the original dissonance between the patient and the interviewer. It looks as though Anthony feels under pressure to follow the interviewer towards feelings about his brother. The pressure might be an invitation to establish a false self. However, something takes them beyond this.

MJ: What are you feeling?

(Pause)

Anthony: I'm just feeling sad. It's not a positive thing. I feel very, very sad.

MJ: Not a buzz?

Anthony: No. *(Pause)* I wish I could cry for him. I couldn't. *(Pause)* I went into a meditation, and when I came out, I knew Emma had had my heart. (p. 56)

The interview then went on to explore the relationship with Emma, an ex-girlfriend.

At the point the interviewer asks the question about Anthony's feelings, he is no longer suggesting things to Anthony. Anthony is relieved of the psychoanalyst's point of view. He suddenly feels sad and begins to think about the disaster that relationships have been for him. The suddenness of this change with the interviewer seems reflected in the suddenness with which his heart was stolen by

Emma. On the surface there had been a rather disjointed flow from mother's memories of his infancy, to his brother's death, to the relationship with Emma. However, the logic of the turn to the relationship with Emma seems once again to refer to the present relationship with the analyst. When the analyst enquires about something the analyst doesn't already know ('What are you feeling?') it is as if Anthony's heart is suddenly stolen – and the reason we can see is that suddenly the analyst is a not-knowing person, and therefore on the same wavelength as Anthony – at last. And Anthony's heart is won!

This clinical material, thus far, speaks to the question of whether meaning has been rendered unconscious, or lost altogether. If there is an answer in Anthony's responses to the psychoanalyst's hunting around for meaning, I am suggesting that a radical change took place when the psychoanalyst asked for emotional meaning, rather than supplied it. The implication would therefore be that the patient searches for a listener who can join him in the state of meaninglessness. He is not looking for his hidden meaning, nor is he willing to absorb any old meaning. He needs someone who can start with not knowing before finding meanings. What the interviewer is beginning to do is to recognise Anthony's handicap, his inability to make meaning, and *how that inability happened.*

Misunderstandings or self-destructiveness

So far, the dissonance between the two world views of analyst and Anthony, and the hole in Anthony's world of meaning, have encouraged sympathy for him, and implied a greater than usual effort on the part of the psychoanalyst to make up for Anthony's problems and the psychoanalyst's own admission of limits to his understanding. However, this sympathy may not be completely justified, as Anthony's self-burning, as well as roasting the psychoanalyst in mocking contempt, suggests a powerful degree of violence in Anthony.

The meaningless state has three possible explanations – meaning is hidden (repressed), or it is missing, or it has been wilfully destroyed. In the third case we need to consider whether there are actual self-destructive attacks on the relevant ego-functions, i.e. attacks on the perceptual apparatus, on alpha-function or on the reality principle.

The next segment of the exploratory interview I want to extract illuminates whether meaning has succumbed to a self-destructive attack on ego-functions. The report of the interview continued with analyst and patient talking about Anthony's love for Emma. He described it as a bad trip with LSD, which he thought was too much for Emma to cope with:

Anthony: That frightened her, that she could have such an effect on someone, and then I burned myself after I saw her for the last time. I set fire to the dance hall. *(Pause)* You know she treated me like her husband, making me cups of tea and looking after me like a wife. There's an awful lot of evidence like that to imply she loved me.

MJ: I see. And after you saw her, you burned yourself?

Anthony: It was just that she got in contact with my love for the world, and I felt I had to do something. It was the day I visited her. I went to the dance hall and started the fires. She knew that. I just went in and lit the fires. I didn't want to kill myself, though.

MJ: What did you want to do?

Anthony: It was a symbolic gesture, the same reason I burned myself in the first place. A gesture to God. I wanted to burn myself inside the building, but I hadn't the guts to do it. It would have been too painful. I just walked out, and the fire-brigade came. (p. 57)

So far, Anthony is working along the lines of the interviewer, trying to understand the events in symbolic terms. The interviewer remains in a mode of enquiry, not-knowing. Anthony in turn is describing his indecision, for or against burning himself to death. But then something else happened:

MJ: It was a symbolic gesture to God, and also connected to having just seen Emma?

Anthony: Yes. It wasn't just seeing Emma, though. My mother was working in the chest clinic at the time, and she got out of the car, and I was getting buzzes from myself that I should burn myself inside the car at the time. I mean, those were absolutely dreadful buzzes. So, so bad. God. So bad. Oh boy. Boy. Christ. *(Becomes distressed)* I was absolutely . . . it was just so bad . . . whole thing was so bad . . . oh . . . oh . . . just living with that all the time, for four years, I can't believe it, it was so bad. (p. 57)

In this sequence Anthony became increasingly distressed. The distress comes off the written page with a force that is probably only a fraction of what it was like in that interview room.

This complete change in the atmosphere of the interview, and the sudden change in Anthony's state of mind, suggest that something had touched him somewhere which neither Anthony nor the interviewer had reckoned with. The interviewer was strongly affected by the explosion of distress, and concluded later:

> the explosion of hatred and perplexity was startling and unexpected. It carried a conviction and authenticity that were in complete contrast with his way of talking up till that point . . . Before the outburst, he had talked in a manner that was patronizing and very much in control of the proceedings. (p. 62)

This moment of change suggests something very specific for Anthony. He had come alive in a most dreadful way. We would be inclined to think that indeed there was a moment of authentic truth somewhere in what had just been said, which drove accurately to some experience or memory that truly existed in Anthony.

Might we accept that there is a psychoanalytic truth in that moment? Might we accept that something hidden endures inside Anthony that responded to a specific image, and to that alone? The indications were that it was something to do with mother in her car, and her leaving it. On this evidence, Jackson formulated at the end of the chapter the dynamics around Anthony's intolerable pain of being left by mother – and by Emma.[6] There was much other evidence to point to this crucial experience of mother; Jackson set out that evidence in his conclusions. The implicit claim, in line with classical psychoanalysis, is that there is something in the patient to be found, revealed and worked upon. There is indeed true meaning here, and as it comes out of hiding, it provokes an outburst of distress. This could be called a psychoanalytic truth, like a scientific discovery of an objective kind.[7]

6 Later it emerged, in therapy after his hospital admission, that he had a memory of mother having a miscarriage when he was not yet three. His guilt and his identification with the dying baby inside mother combined to drive Anthony to die inside the dance-hall.

7 This, as I have said, is debatable. The other side of the debate argues that psychoanalysis is about generating meaning rather than revealing truth. Someone with a

This moment in the interview presents a dilemma for the analyst. Should he pursue his interpretations of missing meaning, or is he now confronted with some other situation that is a crisis, an emergency? In fact, the problem at this moment is not the absence of a coherent meaning, but the absence of a coherent mind.

Interpreting meaning or interpreting ego damage

The interviewer in fact continues by trying to keep the meaning coherent. He tries to go on reconstructing the narrative of Anthony's history:

MJ: Living with the impulse to go into a place and burn yourself.
Anthony: Yes. Oh . . . oh boy . . . I hate that, you know I really hate that *(Shouts, clutches his head, rocks back and forth)* . . . oh . . . how could anybody do that to anybody, you know. I mean who the fuck did that?
MJ: It doesn't feel like you?
Anthony: No, it doesn't.
MJ: A terrible memory, but it's confusion too.
Anthony: Aah . . . yes. I suppose it's confusion . . . oh . . . (pp. 57–58)

hermeneutic viewpoint could argue that the experience of mother leaving is not specific for Anthony. Such an experience is normal enough in the infant's world, and even if it hangs on into adulthood. Therefore, all that was happening was that Anthony and the interviewer between them were constructing a disturbing narrative. The moment of disturbance is not idiosyncratically connected with Anthony, but suddenly Anthony is connected to a plausible general human narrative. It is not that his unconscious has been forced to reveal something; rather a new narrative has been supplied to fill the gap.

However, that argument can be countered. We might point to the unexpectedness of the occurrence. Both patient and interviewer were taken unawares. Jackson was not at that moment looking for anything specific about mother – she just appeared and the outburst erupted. The narrative was not inserted into Anthony's mind by the interviewer. Nor did they jointly construct a coherent narrative of Anthony's experience and problems. Indeed, it did not exist as a coherent narrative for Anthony. Far from it. At that point Anthony was overwhelmed in a manner characterised by incoherence. It was not an epiphany that shocked him; it was something that shattered (or fragmented) his ability to articulate at all. It was not the creation of coherent meaning, but the reverse.

Now the interviewer found himself talking of confusion, instead of eliciting narrative meaning. He was shocked by the eruption, and abandoned narrative in favour of recognising the loss of meaning. Anthony's discourse became fragmented, disjointed words and phrases which in themselves contained very little meaning. Along with the semantic incoherence, there is a powerful emotional impact. Anthony is no longer communicating his thoughts symbolically. The style of communication indicates something of what has happened to Anthony's mind; it seems to have come apart in fragments. The verbal fragments indicate his mental fragmentation. Anthony's mind has lost its coherence and resorts to something more like the expulsion of that state of mind, which then shocks the interviewer's mind. The interviewer was pushed to concede that he must abandon the search for meaning, and stay with the confusion and perplexity. Anthony, in this psychotic moment, reverted to evacuation of particles (exclamations, partial sentences, etc.) and inserted alarm into the psychoanalyst via a concrete transfer of a part of his mind. It is a vivid example of the impact of psychosis on the carer, which we examined in Essay 1.

For Anthony, in shock, hatred is at a distressing height. And that is the moment when the mind is demolished, every bit as much as the hut/dance-hall that he burnt down. Anthony stutters, and stammers, and can only utter 'ohs' and 'aahs'. One feels his inarticulateness painfully. This is a violent process. It conforms to a clinical representation of the self-directed destructiveness of schizoid mechanisms as Klein and her followers described. The mind is split up, as evidenced by the stream of incoherent syllables. More than this, the remnants of words impact concretely on the listener. There is a direct, non-verbal insertion into the analyst, and even into the reader of the account. The distress that has blown Anthony's mind apart at that moment renders words into 'things' that carry distress and have lost their semantic symbolic quality. This conforms to Freud's account of the way words become reduced to things. Or alternatively, words become concrete particles of distress, equated with what they are supposed merely to represent, in line with the account that Segal gave of the psychotic failure of symbol-formation.

In fact, the interviewer does retain some coherence in his thoughts and words, unlike Anthony. He does at least coherently express something of the incoherence, confusion and perplexity. Anthony recovers momentarily. Once the analyst was on the same confused wavelength again, Anthony could regain a degree of coherence and could express something of his state of mind more clearly.

MJ: A terrible memory, but it's confusion too.
Anthony: Aah . . . yes. I suppose it's confusion . . . oh . . . I know I've felt that before, you know. I never felt so much hatred for life for doing that. You know. I feel so much hatred. It was something I could never understand. (p. 58)

Shortly after this, Anthony had to terminate the interview (which was continued at a later point).

After the interviewer could articulate his state as confusion, and terrible, Anthony did recover a capacity to make coherent sentences again. He could make a decision too, to finish the interview.

The non-psychotic and the psychotic parts of the self

We have a moment when a brief acute psychotic process occurred in front of the psychoanalytic observer. It indicates that a conflict developed over separation from mother – and Emma. It became immediately overlaid by severe damage to an ego-function – in this instance, damage to mental coherence and to symbol-formation. There is both conflict and deficit in this. However, whatever the conflict is, the end state is a problem of the ego which requires repair. Bion contrasted the ego's non-psychotic struggle to resolve emotional conflicts (neurosis) with the psychotic ego's need to repair itself. Bion's point is that the non-psychotic deals in meanings, and meaningful communication, while the schizophrenic mind expels experiences.

The contrast between psychotic and non-psychotic mental functioning is demonstrated well by Anthony's change to the mode of expulsion when his speech degenerates into fragments. He transfers distress of such an intensity that it shocks the interviewer and, indeed, perhaps the reader. So, it would appear that Jackson has persistently for most of the assessment interview been speaking, in terms of emotional meanings to a non-psychotic part of Anthony's mind. The indicative moment, because of the intensity of its impact on the psychoanalyst, disrupted his mind from the trajectory he was on, and brought him smartly from discovering meanings to recognising mental (or ego) fragmentation. At that moment the analyst was not able to recognise the process that had happened, only the end result of it: confusion. The psychoanalyst was driven to abandon his rapport with the non-psychotic part of Anthony's mind, and resort to a simple description of the psychotic part. The change highlights the dilemma for a psychoanalyst. The psychotic part is disabled in speech and words; the non-psychotic self is remote from the psychotic problems and intends to keep as remote as possible rather than be overwhelmed. So, which part of the patient should one speak to?

There is not a consensus over how to answer that question.

What model; which intervention?

The way psychoanalysts work derives from the theories they hold. The service that theory can offer is to guide technique in the best direction. It might seem that with such a spread of theories there is a vast selection of methods with which to conduct a psychoanalysis of a schizophrenic. However, this is not exactly the case. Reflections on Murray Jackson's case suggest that the various theories emphasise aspects that interchange with each other in the process of the therapeutic contact. At the start of the interview and also at subsequent points, the couple were struggling with a dissonance in their worlds of meanings. At other times there seemed to be holes, or gaps, in the patient's capacity to articulate or experience; and finally there was an eruption of severe self-destructive violence and hatred, which maimed the patient's mind (temporarily in this case). Study of case material can put the theoretical schools into some relation with each other in a way that a purely conceptual analysis cannot.

It appears from the work of this sensitive analyst, Murray Jackson, that there is always the risk of dissonance between patient and analyst, however sensitive. The technical recommendations of the Sullivanian school may have important practical implications in the conduct of an analysis. There may be important issues of security and survival bound up in the necessary attunement with a schizophrenic patient: a point of view shared by Winnicott. However, it may be exaggerated for Sullivan to base a whole theoretical structure on this clinical observation, and to proclaim this as a basis for the whole course of analysis.

Once a sufficient attunement is established, new phenomena emerge. In Jackson's case, Anthony indicated a loss of ego-function, his silence, i.e. his inability to use words in a way that linked him in communication with mother. We can associate this gap with Lacan's foreclosure of paternal function which leaves a defect in maintaining the boundary functions of a 'paternal' figure, and results in language problems of the kind Freud (1915) described in his essay on the unconscious (words become concrete things).

That problem with boundaries and symbols was also addressed theoretically by Segal, whose theoretical model was different again. She derived the symbolisation problem from a violent attack on the ego's capacity to accept and perceive separation (or boundaries). Interestingly, Jackson's case showed this mind-blowing fragmentation of the ego and its functions – particularly Anthony's function of using words symbolically. However, it was the result of a paroxysm of pain and hatred. It looks as though there is an active self-destructive moment; as Anthony says, a 'hatred for life'.

This exploratory session moved between these three processes. It seems to me that it is not necessarily a regular sequence, but a movement that occurs erratically between them. Nor do I think that this is an exhaustive list of processes. We have covered many more in the survey in this essay. Though the occurrence of these processes may move from one to another, in fact some may be more fundamental than others. It would seem to me that ego-defects are likely to be a 'deeper' factor than interpersonal dissonance; self-destructive attacks are likely to be causal to the effect on verbal symbolisation, and so on. It might lead us to recommend a cautious approach, matching the intervention to whichever particular process is active at the moment – interpersonal or intra-psychic; meaning-generating or meaning-destructive.

This could be one strategy: moving levels, as relevant for the patient. As a result we might need to bear in mind all the possible processes that have been discovered in psychosis – some of which have been summarised in this essay.

There is another, perhaps simpler, strategy: to stay with the deepest layers of process, which always need to be interpreted – for instance, self-destructiveness that underlies ego-deficits.

However, both these strategies are problematic when we come to the process, in schizophrenia, in which words lack symbolic value. Psychoanalytically we are constrained to use words. Perhaps the future research needs to concentrate on how to communicate with an analysand bereft of the capacity to use words reliably. Alternatively, psychoanalysis may need the assistance of psychiatry, where communication with patients is not constrained to words, and where actions may speak louder (Griffiths and Hinshelwood 1997).

There are undecided issues here:

- what language to speak, one of symbols or of actions;
- which part of the patient to speak to, the psychotic or the non-psychotic.

However, these are to do with the psychoanalytic treatment of psychosis, and the argument here is that psychoanalytic understanding is better directed to the psychotic's experience, the impact it has on carers, and the effects on the organisational dynamics of containing psychotic experience. We will now turn to the last of these in Essay 3.

Essay 3

Suffer the mad

Countertransference in the institutional culture

> The lolly scramble was a feature of some days and held both for the amusement of the staff, who often described themselves as 'going dippy ourselves, stuck on duty here all day', and for the pleasure of the patients. The nurses, feeling bored because there hadn't been a recent fight, would fetch a bag of sweets from the tin which was brought every fortnight as part of the Social Security allowance for patients. The paper-lollies would be showered into the middle of the day room and it would be first come first served, with fights developing, people being put in strait-jackets, whistles blowing; and the tension which mounted and reached its peak at intervals both in the patients and in nurses who long ago had had to suppress any desire to 'nurse' and were now overworked, degraded, in many cases sadistic, custodians, found its release, for a while.
>
> (Frame 1962, pp. 86–87)

In this essay, I shall build on the description in Essay 1 of the impact of psychosis on carers. I shall argue that the impact on carers affects the way they relate to the work together, and impacts on institutional care itself.

Reality for psychotic patients has lost its meaning. Since the psychiatric institution and its staff and inmates are the reality for a patient in residence, the institution is an entity without meaning for those patients. It is not surprising that the atmosphere on a ward where psychotic people stay for long periods acquires a sense of no purpose, no meaning. Staff become non-entities for those whom they want to help. A bleak 'belle dame sans merci' atmosphere affects everyone; by and large those institutions have been closed down for their pains. Populated by shuffling figures in ill-laundered, unfitting garb, bent on spending their days measured in cigarette stubs, the silent televisions high on the walls out of arm's reach like gargoyles, the ancient, overcrowded and impersonal dormitories, the silence, the worn-out furniture hardly distinguishable from the figures sitting in it, the old mental hospitals testified to the concentrated doses of lack of meaning and loss of identity. Descriptions cannot exaggerate the depressing impact of the atmosphere in such places, nor therefore the halting dedication of those who went on being carers there (Hinshelwood 1979, 2001).

Not much is now written about institutionalisation, nor the deleterious effects of psychiatric organisation on the recipients of our care. Where such questions are considered they tend to be closed off by received knowledge based on power structures, a Goffmanesque or Foucaultian diatribe about the irresponsible power that the caring professions wield. In this essay I want to raise doubts about that closed question. I want to raise the possibility that the crucial problem for psychiatric institutions is the impact of psychosis and the ensuing anxiety that carers have – not the power they have. It is a somewhat unconventional approach, and this account may seem sketchy.

The power of psychosis renders families, friends and loved ones quite ineffective. So, what happens to those institutions that do *not* give up on psychotic patients? I shall suggest that the distress of the inmates and their carers affects the institution itself. The institution as an entity is consumed by the same psychotic processes – but on a different scale. That is to say the organisation itself subverts meanings, and treats personal identity as a highly impersonal thing. The importance of this line of thinking is that if the work generates personal, interpersonal, and organisational dynamics, they may not be eradicated simply by removing those old institutions. The serious risk is that the same psychiatric problems will impact on us in the community, and the same institutionalising processes will recur in the new institutions set up to deal with psychosis there. Then, fatefully, our new institutions will not recognise such effects because no-one expects them, and all need to deny disillusionment.

'Meaning' and 'identity' are twin casualties of schizophrenia. Psychiatric institutions are the repositories of large quantities of lost meaning and distorted identity. The pragmatic way of dealing with the problem was to close the institutions, level them to the ground and sell for a profit. The really interesting question is not what to do with the end result, but how did it come about? How did all those willing carers and needy patients create only something to be destroyed? How can we know that all our effort to rebuild psychiatry in the community will be buttressed against those old and damaging institutional processes?

From the late 1950s, the introduction of new psychiatric drugs meant that even the least inspiring psychiatrists could begin to let their patients out of the wards. The Mental Health Act in 1957 boosted hopes. The old-fashioned large mental hospitals were predicted to close, and care moved into the community. By 1980, the community had become the focus for psychiatric services. Great effort was made to reorganise services and develop community care units and agencies. After such commitment over recent decades, it takes considerable moral courage to accept that old problems have even now not been faced. Alongside the massive imbalance between recruitment and retention, leading to chronic shortages and long-term vacancies in the psychiatric professions, there is a rather frantic hopefulness. That hope has turned towards drugs, assisted by the well-orchestrated, and well-funded, public relations of pharmaceutical companies. The hope remains precarious, and a more questioning approach towards community psychiatry does not support wild hopes.

In the 1990s concerns about the effectiveness of community care could not be completely concealed. Questions as to whether community care was 'illusion or reality' (Leff 1997), or 'chaos or containment' (Foster and Roberts 1998) began to be asked seriously:

> we are used to thinking of [institutionalisation] as a process that takes place within institutions but [it] can also occur within the community if the mentally ill and their carers are isolated. (Foster 1998, p. 68)

This impression is backed up by figures:

> It is possible for patients to be living in the community but not to be socially integrated with ordinary people . . . To see whether this was the case, we defined a category of social contact, termed an acquaintance, who was involved in neither providing nor receiving psychiatric care. We found that there was an increase in the proportion of patients who knew at least one acquaintance, from 19 per cent in the hospital to 29 per cent in the community . . . It was reassuring to find that some patients had made social

> contact with ordinary members of the public, but they still represent only a small minority of those discharged. (Leff 1997, p. 81)

The result is a degree of de-institutionalisation in community care, but it is a very small effect, and the large majority – over two-thirds – remain socially isolated and in effect institutionalised, now within community care itself.

The isolation of the psychotic is only surprising in the context of psychiatric attitudes towards community care, which remain stoutly optimistic that this is the best solution for people with mental illness. Not enough of these kinds of study, which test the basic claims for abandoning the large mental hospital, have yet been done. Clearly some evidence exists – intuitive and statistical – that institutionalisation was not left behind in the old psychiatric hospitals. More work is needed to demonstrate this conclusively. However, in professional and public opinion, psychiatric patients become isolated and can deteriorate while in the community, in ways that resemble the processes in the old institution. Those that shuffled round our mental hospitals now shuffle along our streets.

Many psychiatrists would claim that the phenomenon of isolation and deteriorating identity is merely an aspect of the long-term affects of schizophrenia. In other words, it is part of the illness, not a product of the institution. This might be substantiated on the grounds that long-standing schizophrenia results from whatever social context. Thus if the social context changes and the condition remains the same, the social context is not a factor. However, this argument, in this simple form, cannot be responsibly sustained. First, the argument could only validly conclude that a social factor is not the *sole* causal one. It does not rule out other factors, which may of course coexist with the social ones. Second, alarmingly, the argument could lead to the view that closing the large hospitals – because institutions are bad for patients – was never valid. Third, intuitive conclusions of this kind (that 'institutionalisation' results from the schizophrenia) need more consideration, because after all, the need for the hospital closure programme was a similar intuitive conclusion, and it behoves us not to jump to obvious conclusions.

What I shall attempt to do in this essay is to give a different account. It is an account of the problems that psychiatric institutions have precisely because they house schizophrenic patients – whether the large obsolete old hospitals, or the new community care agencies.

Essay 1 described the impact of psychosis on carers. That process, started by the illness, is completed by the social context. Psychiatric carers are organised in a social entity that is affected by the psychology of the carers. Their disturbance affects the culture and then the functioning of the service they are all part of. The impact, unconscious as it often is, leads to unconscious features of the interpersonal system. The most large-scale is 'schism', in which the organisation divides into separate camps with different sets of attitudes to the work and to each other. This division is common in the psychiatric services – exemplified by the contest between the biological and psychological systems of explaining mental health and organising the work. The biological approach, usually regarded as a scientific approach, has an increasing dominance in contemporary psychiatry in many countries. That approach has specific attitudes towards the work, and is supported by influences within and outside psychiatry. Its dominance tends to make it seem the approach of psychiatry as a whole. The set of attitudes in turn affects patients, determines treatments and skews outcomes in our services. Other attitudes towards the work and towards patients tend to be excluded rather than incorporated. In so far as those attitudes downplay subjective experience, they too are responsible for the neglect of the psychology of carers – one of the motivations for the thinking in this book.

Unconscious interpersonal systems

For the individual, the institution is a variegated and structured object. It offers complex opportunities to play out issues in the way a child plays out issues, with her toys in a playroom. As Jaques summarised:

> Individuals may put their internal conflicts into persons in the external world, unconsciously follow the course of the conflict by means of projective identification. (Jaques 1955, pp. 496–497)

At the level of the unconscious, persons relate to each other at work in terms of fundamental issues and conflicts which are displaced into problems with achieving the work task, and into the culture of the organisation. Depending on how the external situation evolves, they:

> re-internalise the course and outcome of the externally perceived conflict by means of introjective identification. (Jaques 1955, p. 497)

So, the individual perceives the external world in her own terms. She sees her own issues developing there and may see them resolved in the interaction between others. There is a very concrete quality to this. Colleagues and patients may actually become the embodied version of her own imaginings and unconscious phantasies. At the same time, they have to be colleagues in achieving the *conscious* task. A degree of tension between the real work and the unconscious issues must creep in. Because of its partially unconscious nature, the tension is hard to pin down and deal with. In psychiatric work, where unconscious phantasies are intense, there is scope for very powerful interference with the conscious task. Richard Davies (1996) described an illustration of this, which I summarise:

> A disturbed man had a harsh mother as a child. She was violent and humiliated him. When released from prison where he had finished a sentence for brutal sexual crimes, he asked to be kept inside. The request was naturally refused. Later he went to a police station with a similar request, and was similarly rejected. He subsequently engaged with the helping network in a specific way. That network responded disastrously to his continuing disturbance. He was dangerous and a specific plan was set out at his hostel to ensure that only male staff dealt with him. The arrangements quickly broke down for extraneous reasons. He was taken into intensive counselling by a female worker; and a female prison visitor who had visited him in prison continued to see him, including taking him to her home, where he assaulted her. Another female worker offered counselling, sometimes in evening sessions, and afterwards said she had forgotten that he was a rapist! The staff did not seem to realise the danger he posed, and the breakdown of the precautionary arrangements.
>
> What went wrong could be traced very specifically to a repetition of the experience of care the man had as a child. His mother was very powerful and controlling and continually made him feel powerless; he effectively had no father with whom to identify. His sense of maleness was unpractised and uncontrolled. In the hostel, the male staff disappeared – changed job, or went on

> courses. Unthinkingly, the female staff let themselves be drawn into taking up powerful professional roles with him. They were inviting to him, and then withdrew, giving him that intolerable feeling of powerlessness again.

The staff seemed unable any longer to think about the client realistically, or even to remember his case fully. A fairly simple professional insight – that his violent and humiliating criminal activity was connected with violence and humiliation he received from his mother – seemed to become unusable.

Davies arouses our concern that the evident wish on the man's part to receive some sort of help for his internal state was not 'read' by the helpers, and he progressed to further violent crimes, one of which was the assault on the female helper. There was a problem in 'reading' the plea for help. The staff were sucked into playing out roles in the patient's inner and past life. The whole episode lacked an articulate meaning, and the staff lost their professional competence. The unconscious playing-out of this man's powerful internal issues interfered with the minds and work of the trained professionals. They carried out their *conscious* tasks, apparently unaware of how affected they were by this man's conflicts, and their part in playing them out. Such dramatisation, by staff, of the inner worlds of those in the institution is a very common (but unrecognised) phenomenon (Hinshelwood 1987a).

These carers became caught in the intra-psychic 'play' of the person they cared for. The deeply personal past, in which the man was trapped, came to be represented in actual terms by the present selection of people. The women in the team became embodiments of the mother who caused such humiliation. This was predicted, consciously, but, because of unconscious forces, professional prediction changed to unconscious enactment without the staff realising how they had forgotten the prediction, and the professional task. The man's demand was treated with a 'care' response, but not a reflective, articulated one. It was a sentimentalised sympathy, which passed as maternal caring, but in the event recapitulated his experience of maternal humiliation. Neither the man nor the carers were able to articulate what was happening. Proper symbolisation, conscious representation, and thought failed to survive. His request to stay in prison, for instance, was treated as meaningless by the prison authorities, and no doubt consciously by the man himself. The recognition that the man's 'self-control' had to be taken over and embodied by others (similar to the admission of a psychotic patient to a mental hospital, described in Essay 1, 'Responsibility and professional identity', p. 12) had been lost in this community care case.

Who was in control? The power relations are much more complex than a naïve Foucaultian view (see Hinshelwood 1997). In fact, the man's own demands were the more powerful, and overwhelmed the professional probity of the workers. The admission of a psychiatric patient to hospital is forced upon the service, yet they are forced to *be* his self-control. So it was with this patient in the community. For instance, the man asked the prison to go on performing the role of his self-control for him. The police were also invited. The refusal of the prison and police to comply with that need for control was technically a precise observance of their responsibilities. Processes of complex interchange of initiative and agency, responsibility and identity, lead to caricature stereotypes of staff and patients (Hinshelwood 1998), as we saw in Essay 1 ('Institutionalisation', p. 13).

Meaning can only be reconstructed by an observer taking the kind of distanced overview that Richard Davies was able to take. The service played out an apparently insightless drama. Meaning was lost in the unthinking action, and clarity of thought diminished in both parties. Carers became lost in *being parts of his drama*, rather than being themselves. Their thoughtful, trained professional selves capsized under the interpersonal processes, and a primitive violent play was unconsciously instituted instead.

This is an instance of an organisational process in which interpersonal relations redistribute experiences and even parts of the individuals through the social network. The interest of Davies' example is that such an institutional process of redistribution of experiences can occur in a community care setting. That process can occur in a repeated way in long sequences so that parts of persons and their experiences move as if in independent motion around the organisation. In one example (see Hinshelwood 1989a), a quarrel that frustrated a doctor was passed through various staff to end up in a staff meeting that was eventually moved to deal with an institutional problem. So, one person's individual experience was depersonalised by the progressive interchange between people. Some 'thing' appeared to pass around, leading to an eventual conversion into an institutional decision. These are projective and introjective steps in sequence. They affect the identity of the individuals and their experiences of themselves and of others. In the course of this step-by-step process the emotional activity moves from the level of an individual to one that is an interaction between individuals, and eventually to group activity, cultural assumptions, and institutional action. Something of the person is swept away into group and institutional activity. (Detailed illustrations can be found in Hinshelwood 1989a, 1989b); these serial cycles of projection and introjection that result in long sequences in the institutional network are explored more fully in Hinshelwood (2001). The character of this depersonalising process leads to the familiar experience of institutions as impersonal and faceless. In a way, such processes are quite ordinary, and we can see ourselves in them, and the effects of most institutions. At the same time they represent the strangest occurrences affecting our identity. These unconscious processes run concurrently with the actual task. We can speak of the:

> phantasy form and content of an institution [that] refer to the form and content of social relationships at the level of the common individual phantasies which the members of an institution share by projective and introjective identification. (Jaques 1955, p. 482)

They give rise to identities or roles in the organisation that derive from phantasy life, and that shape our institutions in hidden ways.

Disorders of the task

Under the pressure of such unconscious phantasies, the task changes in certain ways. For instance, in the last example the task of containing this violent man in a hostel drifted to one of providing maternal care in a thoughtless and somewhat sentimentalised way. 'Task drift' is a common distortion of the task, and involves the characteristic distortion of professional identity (Menzies 1979). Another common distortion is where the task drifts in two different directions in different parts of the organisation.

Distortions of the task are one effective way of spotting unconscious institutional pathology of this kind (Miller and Rice 1967). Distortion occurs when there is uncertainty about the task, and suggests some motivated uncertainty about the task. Uncertainty may occur where there are multiple tasks that have to be carefully prioritised,[1] and particularly when tensions and unconscious conflicts are high. These problems are also particularly frequent when there is inadequate discussion on the task priorities. In psychiatric institutions, unfortunately, there are reasons why such open discussion cannot properly take place. I address the super-ego manifestations within the culture of care in Essay 1 ('The professional super-ego', p. 22).

Task drift

In place of the uncertainties, conflicts and confusion, new tasks can be implicitly substituted that have the advantage that they give more certainty and they simplify conflicts. For instance, Menzies described a residential school for disturbed children. The children

1 In our services that care for those who are most disturbed, we may have an inherent uncertainty as to the task that is required of us (Spillius 1976). Those who are most uncontainable by the family, or by friends and neighbours, must be contained by the psychiatric service, taking over from family, friends and neighbours. We must cope where they could not. So, we function not just for the patient who wants an asylum, where reality can be neglected; we must also satisfy the family and relatives etc. by incarcerating the patient in a custodial confinement, so that society will no longer have to withstand the impact of psychosis. Our institutions and services exist to care for patients, and also to spare relatives. In addition, carers have been increasingly led to think of themselves as offering treatment with the expectation that they will cure or at least ameliorate the disease. These contrasting expectations placed on the institution are not all compatible, and therefore staff feel the strain of expectations pulling them in different directions (see Spillius 1976). Three tasks compete:

- patients want asylum;
- relatives want the patient incarcerated away from them;
- staff want to treat as medical and nursing professionals.

Staff have to perform mixtures of these incompatible tasks, and they can become confused. For example, nurses can come to represent the custodial side, despite their care role; similarly, doctors may devote themselves to treatments despite having to be responsible for compulsory detention of patients. Both doctors and nurses may have to press patients to take their treatments, such as tablets or ECT, while confronting the patient's demands to be left alone and relieved of ordinary human responsibilities. These various and conflicting tasks are not easy to handle.

Mediating the variable primacy of tasks in such institutions is no easy responsibility and calls for frequent decisions about moment-to-moment primacy at all levels in the organisation, often without adequately defined managerial policy (Menzies 1979, p. 198).

were deprived, and aroused the teachers' wish to become better 'parents' than the children had previously had. This conflicted with the educational task of the school. In this case, the teachers had diminished the conflict by implicitly redefining the task to one of care and need-gratification rather than learning. The care aspect of the work surely does exist in that kind of educational institution, but it cannot have priority on a regular basis. When the school task moved from education to gratifying dependency, the staff role changed from teacher to carer. As a result, different aspects of the teachers' conduct were valued and different ones looked down on. A strict line on homework, for instance, might be valued in a teaching task, but once the school drifted to the task of care, strictness about homework could become disapproved of as harsh. As the task drifted from teaching to dependency gratification, the professional role changed from an identity as a teacher to one as a surrogate parent.

The task of an organisation is therefore vulnerable, subject to conflict, confusion, implicit redefinition, and drift. These task problems occur more in institutions where there is an actual conflict of primacy in the institution's social task, and where there is a diminished capacity in the institution for adequate reflection on what the task is and should be. Shortly we will consider a third very important problem with the task, beyond confusion and drift. This is schism, where the task drifts in two separate directions. Then there is no conflict in the task, just a conflict between different sub-groups of staff.

Culture and task

These problems with the task are often difficult to grapple with. They are not problems with the machinery (e.g. the ECT apparatus needs servicing) nor with structural aspects of the organisation (e.g. how many nurses should be on duty at night time). They have to do with something more ephemeral: the attitudes to the work. These are internal features of the members of a team, yet they are co-ordinated in some unspecified way among a team of staff. Eric Trist (1950/1990) talked of the need for a psychosocial concept, one which expressed this bridge between the personal on one hand and the social on the other. He pointed to social attitudes held in common by individuals as such a psychosocial phenomenon. He referred to it as culture. The culture includes many things,[2] but typically a 'belief system' holds the members of a society together in a single culture. Beliefs are commonly held attitudes that embody values of a positive or negative kind. Individuals hold attitudes and beliefs by virtue of their membership of a social group and its culture; attitudes and beliefs are implicit certificates of membership of the group. A social culture provides:

> the complex of mental attitudes, implicit as well as explicit, that a person needs to hold in order effectively to live, work and communicate within his human collective. (Miller and Gwynne 1972, p. 88)

In the particular context we are considering here, the belief system is a collection of attitudes and values about the work, and the task that is held to be primary in the work.

How the co-ordination of beliefs, attitudes and values occurs is a matter of group dynamics. In a group, separate individuals, each with his or her individual views, background and motives, come to have an allegiance to attitudes held in common by all the group members. For instance, doctors tend to think of themselves as highly educated and the people best 'in the know' about each patient – a view not necessarily shared by nurses. Jon Stokes (1994) used Bion's theories of basic assumptions to characterise the interdisciplinary rivalries among the psychiatric professions (Bion 1961). Doctors tend to promote dependency attitudes, therapists (or nurses perhaps) a collusive pairing, and social workers a semi-paranoid fight on behalf of the patient. Stokes argued that difficulty with the primary task enhances the basic assumptions and attitudes to the work (primitive dependency, pairing or fight–flight), which sets the different disciplines against each other. These separate emotional understandings of the task give a different 'feel' or atmosphere to the culture of each profession.

2 Raymond Williams (1958) has given a full account of the meandering meaning of the term through history. Roger Scruton (1983) indicates that culture is composed of 'activities which embellish and colour the process of survival, and give it its distinctive local forms', and thus consists of 'customs, habits of association, religious observances, even specific beliefs'. My sense of the word in a psychiatric context emphasises the *unconscious* attitudes and beliefs about the work, i.e. about its forms of practice and about the persons who are the raw material.

Implicitly, my account indicates that some of the social belief system is unconscious and is under the influence of the anxieties and defences typically observed by psychoanalysts. Psychiatric institutions are beset by intense anxieties, and their cultural attitudes to the task are therefore a prey to unconscious psychodynamics at the level of the social group. The task of the psychiatric service – to care for disturbed patients – demands various technologies, groupings and relations, and these will be infected by unconscious pressures arising from the anxieties of the work. All forms of work have some emotional aspects, and give rise to anxiety of some kind among employees. The particular anxiety will depend on the nature of the work. For instance, the technology of a munitions factory must give rise to apprehension about personal safety; caring for terminally ill patients gives intense feelings of concern, frustration and thoughts of death; mining coal is believed to be dangerous; schools make teachers responsible for the whole of young lives; soldiers in the army face death; and so on.

Clearly, the psychiatric culture has a set of beliefs about its work, about the nature of madness, what it is, what to do about it, control it or cure it, and so on. Moreover, some attitudes embedded in its culture are psychoanalytically unconscious. What is unspoken, hidden or unconscious cannot be adequately spoken and so is most troublesome to manage as an organisation. Unconscious beliefs about the task are significant and contribute strongly to, or interfere with, achieving the task. Roles people play in the work become professional identities which derive from the task influenced by the unconscious beliefs.

Schisms

Organisations that deal with human beings frequently show a specific feature: different aspects of the institution hold different beliefs about the task. There is in effect a cultural schism, meaning that two different belief systems coexist although the different sets of attitudes to what the task is, and the different values given to each version of the task, are held by different people. The division is a way of dealing particularly with conflicts inherent in the task, and ambivalent feelings deriving from the conflict. Then the two sides of the conflict, with separate sides of the ambivalence, separate out as two sub-groupings in the organisation.

A particularly clear example of schism was described by Miller and Gwynne (1972) when they looked at the organisation of the group of Cheshire Homes for the permanently physically disabled. The homes cared for people who would never get better, and could only achieve a quality of life up to a degree allowed by their handicap. The culture of these institutions tended to become one or other of two complementary kinds. The emotional tension was concern for people with both a severe disability and a surviving hope.

On one hand, some were motivated by liberal attitudes. They believed that, however disabled, everyone has some abilities and these can be made use of – some esoteric skill, like painting with a toe. This led to a kind of care in which the inmates were regarded as having a full human potential that merely had to be realised by the staff and brought out. So these homes pressed the individuals to a full development. This was termed by Miller and Gwynne, ironically, the 'horticultural' model. A contrasting paternalistic attitude was held by other homes. They regarded the inmates as deeply damaged and with little chance of achieving any human characteristics. They were there, in the home, to be looked after until such time as the biological death caught up with the social one. This pressure on inmates towards becoming inert recipients of scrupulously dutiful care was termed the 'warehousing' model.

In both kinds of homes, horticultural and warehousing, there was genuine concern for the inmates. Staff sincerely wished to do the best that could possibly be done for them. But in both cases 'care' was reduced to one aspect of care, with the exclusion of another. The horticultural model denied the full handicap of the inmate and a full humanity was proclaimed – with ultimate distress to many who couldn't paint with a single toe. In the warehousing culture, a paternalism overlooked any surviving potential and talent, in the belief that inmates needed total care, and this led to many leading lives that were unnecessarily restricted.

Here the care of the severely physically damaged and handicapped was divided across a fracture line. The handicapped are not capable of normal life; nor are they necessarily completely devoid of skills and potential. The damage and the surviving potential are two aspects of each individual. They call out very different feelings from the staff. The exact proportion of each individual needs to be assessed in every case, and repeatedly assessed over time. But the confluence of these two – damage and potential, coinciding in the same person – is a painful realisation for both inmates and staff. Sadness and hope coexist with uncommon intensity, and tear the heart in two. Because of that pain, staff (and inmates as well) separate the sets of attitudes and, in the process, separate the feelings. So, inmates in some homes are believed to be only damaged; whereas in others they are only full of potential. In this way two different realities are constructed, and that results in less immediate pain. However, each reality is distorted, and that unnecessarily distorts the life of the inmates, as well as the job satisfaction of the staff. In the longer term, distress is generated in the process of alleviating it.

Using my own experience when working in a prison where I was a visiting psychotherapist during the 1970s, I came to see the defensive techniques that operated in the culture (Hinshelwood 1993). The prison officers, as well as the prisoners, operated sets of practices that derived from quite different attitudes to the task of the prison.

> The anxiety the officers felt was a fear of violence. On the other hand, the prisoners were emotionally threatened by an overwhelming unconscious guilt. The prison system co-ordinated the practices of officers and prisoners to support defensiveness against the specific anxieties.
>
> The practices supported defensive attitudes. The officers asserted the value of strength and toughness, manifested in the ordered rituals of locking and controlling. This was aimed at managing their fear of violence, and supported a belief that all was under control and could not be disturbed. The prisoners' belief system also prized strength, brutality and trickery. However, their version of toughness obliterated any sensitivity that might bring guilt. It was supported by anxious claims of innocence, and it viewed prison officers, police and others as loaded with guilt instead of themselves. So, both officers and prisoners asserted toughness and ruthlessness as the prime virtues in this male prison, sought to demonstrate these features in themselves, and used others to do so.
>
> One means open to both officers and prisoners to sustain their attitudes of toughness was to identify others within the prison system who could be thought of as weak, gullible and guilty. For the prisoners there were certain categories – Pakistanis, sex abusers – who were relegated to this category. For the officers there were certain categories of staff – prison visitors, psychotherapists, women staff – who were defined as weak and soft, and in need of protection from the prisoners' brutality and trickery. These staff groups formed a counter-culture, and held

> different attitudes to the dominant toughness and brutality. Their attitudes were of a more caring kind. But in the eyes of the dominant culture of the prison, caring attitudes were exaggerated as over-trusting, acquiescing and foolishly gullible. Carers represented the polar opposite to the toughness of the dominant culture.

It appeared that the culture was carefully divided into those defined as tough and those defined as weak. The culture of the whole prison contained both these immiscible subcultures, each adhering to a different one-dimensional view – toughness or weakness. These attitudes were necessarily distorted; the tough attitudes lacked concern, and the weak ones lacked firmness. This division of attitudes obstructed the work of a prison in trying to integrate firm control with human concern. The tension between control of the prisoners' criminality and concern at the inhumanity of incarceration was lost in the schismatic separation. Too easily in society – and in the prisons themselves – such tension is avoided by adopting lopsided attitudes: only toughness which becomes repressive, or only concern which becomes sentimental.

Psychiatric cultures

In the psychiatric services, there is also evidence of a deep divide. The staff culture in a mental hospital is divided into opposing sets of attitudes – one dominant set, and one counter-culture (Hinshelwood 1994b). Somewhat like the prison, the divided culture appears to be organised to cope with all those anxieties that come from the work – in this case, facing madness. The anxieties are somewhat similar for staff and patients, and concern the impact of psychosis (Essay 1). Madness has a specific quality of terror for human beings, and the fear of it is probably managed in various ways by different people. However, collectively in a mental hospital, the individuals seem to develop defensive techniques, as in a general hospital described by Menzies (1959; see also Hinshelwood and Skogstad 2000). Together the staff and patients avoid their fear. This avoidance is based on the attitude that madness comes from intimate emotional contact with others. If anything comes to life in the interaction between people, it will bring madness to life as well. Realistic or otherwise, this belief result in the wards of a mental hospital being run in a particular way, as if everyone proceeds on the basis of that unconscious assumption.

Any liveliness that might go on between people will lead to madness breaking out. Consequently liveliness must be snuffed out quickly, for fear of the predicted madness. Donati (1989) reported observations made on a long-stay ward, and described a characteristic feature of interaction between staff and patients – a 'touch and go' technique, she called it (see also 'The need to care' in Essay 1, p. 23). Often a brief question or greeting to a patient was immediately followed by a closing-off of contact, maybe a physical movement away, or the dismissal of the patient's response. It is to be observed in the minimal contact between patients too. Contact is not completely absent, but is a shallow, concrete and transient moment – like the constant corridor exchanges of cigarettes. The result is a continual blighting of the sense of contact and community in the ward. The consequence is the overpowering quality of deadness in the culture on those wards. The denigration of contact is part of the desperation when contact with psychosis is felt. This cultural belief system is unconscious, but often staff try *consciously* to make the wards more lively (Donati 1989; Hinshelwood 1987b). Because the cause of deadness is not a conscious one, the efforts to remedy the culture become rather hopeless.

However, there is another important aspect of mental hospital life. Although the dominant culture views life, and a depth of contact with patients, as dangerous, a belief in life is re-found elsewhere. There are people working in mental hospitals who proclaim the importance of emotional contact with patients. As in the prison, the disowned and denigrated human concern is exported into certain marginal groups of staff. Among the professional groups, there are those who do represent a personal contact with patients – the expressive therapists, for instance; the psychotherapists; the occupational therapists; the clergy. These people are also on the whole kept at the margins, because they unconsciously represent just that danger which the dominant cultural attitudes believe will trigger madness.

This culture has split in two. On one side, close emotional contact is believed to cause madness, and that attitude leads to work practices (defensive techniques) that avoid personal closeness. On the other side, there is a demand that more closeness is the essence of human experience and the only real chance of therapeutic recovery. Thus two groups are driven towards conflicting one-dimensional attitudes: all closeness is dangerous; closeness is the only hope. Neither side is completely correct. A balanced view might be that closeness is important but has to be judged carefully with each vulnerable person. It is not easy to balance the different aspects of the task. (Barrett (1996, see Essay 1, 'Meaninglessness and understanding', p. 15) described these two sets of attitudes separated in time in terms of different phases in the treatment of each patient.)

Psychiatry and psychoanalysis

This schism in psychiatry is not new. The best part of a century ago, one authority wrote:

> Psychiatry does not employ the technical methods of psychoanalysis; it omits to make any inferences from the *content* of the delusion, and, in pointing to heredity, it gives us a very general and remote aetiology instead of indicating first the more special and proximate causes. But is there a contradiction, an opposition in this? Is it not rather a case of one supplementing the other? (Freud 1917c, p. 254)

Given such a long-standing division between such natural bedfellows, we need to reflect on why they resist coming together. The simple and conscious answer is that they have different rational views on mental disorders and their causation. One turns to biology; the other turns towards the *experiences* of the mental ill:

> Psychoanalysis cannot but cause disquiet to those material scientists who believe that their field of inanimate matter and their methods forged in the study of inanimate matter must form *the* ultimate field and the final method for all science, even that of animate creatures. To hold that science must ultimately be concerned only with inanimate matter is certainly both fashionable and popular, even though this belief may do serious injustice to nature and to the range of science itself. One frequently hears statements such as, 'That's the scientific side – but what about the human side?' as if this latter were not available for science, as if such human matters such as envy, ambition, contentment, play, tenderness were not to be thought of as fit for scientific understanding but were to be put *a priori* beyond the scientific pale. It needs emphasis that this view of science as concerning only hardware, things but not creatures, physics and chemistry, but not people, is curiously seductive. (Main 1967, p. 169)

This suggests that we are seduced into believing in the radical difference between psychoanalysis and 'scientific' psychiatry. My argument has been that it is seductive because people are driven apart under the pressure of dealing with the distress that is inherent in the job psychiatry does. Main's view that 'science' involves objectifying the field of study fits with the dominant attitude in psychiatry, which demands an emotional distance from the disturbance that is the field of study. That simplification is seductive because it reduces the stress arising from the impact of psychosis, described in Essay 1.

I shall illustrate this phenomenon of the two psychiatric subcultures driven into opposition with a piece of consultation, which showed the restriction of thinking on both sides of the schism. In this illustration, a worker represents one side of a professional conflict that exists in the emotional aspects of the work.

> The Worker, trained in psychoanalytic psychotherapy, was employed in a community mental health service. Part of the service was a Therapeutic Milieu (TM) in a Day Centre. Twenty-five psychotic patients were rehabilitated there, if possible, back to the community. The rest of the Centre was a psychiatric out-patient service. In her expert function, the Worker advised on the original setting-up of the TM. In fact, with one of the occupational therapists, she had proposed and fought for the TM in the first place. She had clear ideas about it, and was supportive to the team of less experienced professionals (two occupational therapists, one-and-a-half nurses, one social worker, one work organiser) who ran it now. There were various activities – outings, cooking, therapy, etc. – for those patients able to engage in them. The Worker emphasised the 'dining room'. Patients who could not engage might go to the dining room and sit, supervised by one member of staff. The Worker felt that this area where patients would be free of pressure, and could 'do nothing', was very important. She knew, however, how difficult it was for the staff member to be with them while they did nothing.
>
> The Worker also suggested having a staff meeting on Friday afternoon. The staff could share with each other and reflect on the experiences and any distress they felt from patients' difficulties during the week. Friday was important, as the staff and patients left for the weekend. She herself supervised this group, her only ongoing involvement with the TM once it had been set up. She was careful to limit her direct involvement to this group.

However, it was clear that in setting up the TM she had had a very strong input, and now felt protective of it.

The Friday afternoon group was presented at the consultation session. On the whole it worked well and certain incidents were described. One woman patient had her baby taken into care by the social services, and the staff – especially the contact person (key worker) – felt great distress for the patient and did not know what to do beyond being with her. On another Friday, they had talked about a schizophrenic patient who had been shot in the head. His paranoid state had been confirmed in a most terrifying way. One of the staff members visited him in hospital where he was connected to a lot of tubes and machines, which distressed the staff member considerably.

The Worker described the pressure this staff member felt. Staff wished to find something they could do for patients in distressing situations. The Worker was very good at helping the staff to remain with the patients, without becoming intrusively active. That is to say, they attempted to value the *internal* activity involved in being with the patients and 'doing nothing'.

She presented this work because a disastrous problem had arisen. The authorities in the wider psychiatric service had developed doubts about the TM. Patients stayed too long. Half of the first group of admissions to the TM were still attending three years later. It had been an important principle that the Worker had laid down at the outset that patients should proceed at their own pace. The authorities now decided differently. Patients should be divided in two – those that could be helped and should have a time limit of six months; and those that could not benefit, who should leave and go to other services. Moreover, supervision (of the staff) should be provided by someone from outside the service altogether – pushing out the Worker from her Friday group and from her project.

She was particularly incensed by this interference with her own baby, as it were; the unkindest cut was that she should be relieved of her supervision (the Friday group) in three months' time. The members of her supervision group were equally outraged. The Worker wanted to intervene and join the staff in fighting these decisions. She thought, however, that if she joined in their protest she would be breaking the boundary of supervision and colluding, as it were, with the staff she was supervising. This was the problem she brought.

What was remarkable in this presentation was how often the value of 'doing nothing' was repeated: (a) there was the dining room area which was protected for vulnerable and new patients to 'do nothing'; (b) there was the week's distress contained in the Friday afternoon group which could reflect on the importance of internal 'doing', and simply being with the distressed and distressing patients and avoiding any intrusive 'doing to' them; and (c) there was the Worker's belief that she should do nothing about the authorities' decisions, because if she did it would be 'colluding'. In a way, the manner in which this Worker had helped the staff to see the value of their reflective, internal activity, and had supported them in this, was impressive. Her very success at this made it very poignant that her work was suddenly and brutally being curtailed. It made one want to fight her cause too. This difficult, poignant and taxing work seemed devalued by insightless and unfeeling authorities. In this community service there seemed to be a harsh and stark contrast between speedy treatment on one hand, and reflection ('doing nothing'), on the other. Moreover, that contrast had degenerated into a conflict.

So, the striking features are as follows. A conflict has divided two sets of people: the 'active' authorities who want to foster a throughput in the TM, on one hand; and the reflective Worker with her group who valued 'doing nothing', on the other. These are polarised attitudes that reinterpret care in two opposite directions. Each set of attitudes has become rather extreme and in the process one-dimensional. The sensitivity of the active authorities appears very depleted, and the political energy of the reflective Worker is blocked. This is a schism between cultural sets of attitudes.

However, the divergence between the attitudes of activity and 'doing nothing' corresponds to another similar schism that can be seen in this consultation. A tension exists in the Friday supervision group itself. This is presented as the need to 'be with' the distress of the distressing patients on one hand, and the wish to 'do something' for them on the other. The Worker was very alive to the conflict between the two attitudes *within* the staff. They felt impelled to do something to relieve the patients' distress, and at the same time they valued the *internal* work of simply 'being with' them. The conflict in the TM staff corresponded strikingly with the organisational conflict that had expressed itself *between* people (between the authorities and the Worker). Though they struggled with the internal tension in the supervision (the Friday afternoon group), it had been *partly* avoided (defended against) by a splitting process and they projected the urge to 'do something' into other groupings of the organisation: into the authorities, in fact. As an inter-group dynamic it had become simpler and more straightforward, though hardly more soluble, by being externalised in this way. Internally, individuals were reduced to either one side or the other – doing nothing, or simplistic activity – and in the process they were spared their conflict. The members of the TM staff could split off that wish to do something, and then listen to it being spoken by the authorities who wished for movement and speed. Consciously the staff disagreed with an active approach, but unconsciously they could not help wanting it as well. It appeared that the external authorities had internalised an 'active' mode of being, which in a similar manner simplified any conflict by abolishing reflection (internal activity) and empathy. This was the picture gained by myself as consultant, which I then articulated.

> There was an interesting response from the Worker to this formulation. She looked a bit troubled by the suggestion that she, and her colleagues, unconsciously split off wishes to 'do something'. Then, she described with some bitterness an attitude she found in herself in other parts of her work in the service. She said it led to a certain degree of acting-out. She conducted psychotherapy in the outpatient part of the Centre, but she did not go to the clinical conferences because of the strong active treatment approach (of a biological kind) continually being promoted by the psychiatrists who held authority in the Clinic.
>
> Her reserved non-compliance is understandable in a service with an organised split of this kind. But her own decision not to go to these conferences dramatised the splitting, and must be a contribution to institutionalising it. It put an actual geographical distance between her *reflective* approach and the dominant *active* treatment, through the distance she maintained between herself and the psychiatrists' meeting. 'Reflecting' and 'treating' could only exist if split widely apart. They could clash badly if brought into the same room. When the situation was described thus, the Worker was in fact very alive to it. She could think about a possible element of acting-out in her own professional conduct with the psychiatrists. She looked quite disheartened, though enlightened.

This organisation had divided in a schism between unrealistic stereotypes: first the active carers who do not have a place for reflection, and second the reflectors who are so committed to 'doing nothing' that they cannot act when necessary.

> Interestingly, there was a wider context to this supervision. This Centre was a part of the community care of a large psychiatric service connected to a university hospital. There, evidence of a very prominent and similar splitting between vigorous time-limited methods and reflective psychological attitudes (verging on the timeless) was present. It was those active attitudes that seeped into the authorities' decision to change the TM.

The polarised parts of the system – TM versus biological psychiatry (or the therapeutic worker versus the outpatient psychiatrists) – seem to have both lost something. Each set of attitudes and ideas about the nature of care had become undiscussed and unchallenged, and implicit to each group. These sets of ideas could be called 'ideologies', if that term is taken to mean the inflation of some idea to an overblown importance, with the diminishing of other, perhaps, complementary, ideas. At a level of feelings, there is a primitive separation. The minds of the members of the organisation became located between the two differing groups. Projection and introjection within the network of group relations results in the individuals' losing aspects of themselves and enhancing others by acquisition from another group. Because of the primitive quality of this transmission of feeling states, ordinary dialogue and debate cannot occur. Non-communicating retreat from each other is the only way of coexisting, as when the Worker avoided going to the outpatient meeting. Serious barriers to communication grow up and are acted out. This greatly hampers the work of the organisation as a whole. When encounter does then happen, there is inexplicable friction, which leads either to stalemate or to a fierce domination of one party over the other.

The consultation illustrated how individuals' emotional conflicts in the work are invested in a schism within the organisation. So, organisational schism is important psychologically for the individual. It supports the defence mechanism of splitting that relieves tension *within* him or her. Such an organisational schism connects with, reflects and resolves psychological splitting within individuals. Its purpose is to protect people against painful tensions and conflicts within themselves over the work.

There appear to be two rules that apply to cultural schisms between sub-groups.

1 Internal tensions *within* people become external conflicts *between* people. In the illustration, the psychiatric service subdued a tension between reflecting and acting by separating the two functions into separate groups of people. We might call this *the rule of externalisation.*
2 Sub-groups related to each other develop mutual, complementary distortions. Having separated out, the two psychiatric sub-groups exhibited distorted functions; those representing reflection were at risk of becoming paralysed, while those representing action risked being impetuous. This might be called *the rule of opposites.*

This model for considering organisational function has heuristic value in consulting to organisations or to sub-groups within organisations. When hearing about *this* group conflict, one must bear in mind some other silent internal conflict; when hearing about *this* unit or department, one must bear in mind some *other* unit or department which is at another pole.

Care as culture

The dominant culture in psychiatry holds that distance from the humanity of the psychotic patient is necessary and that a scientific objectivity is all-important. This has some advantage in protecting staff from the impact of psychosis, and indeed offers advantages to the psychotic patient as well (his retreat from reality into asylum). The complementary 'counter-culture' (including psychotherapy, psychoanalysis, and the expressive art and music therapies) is not always therapeutically beneficial either. The central tenet of the counter-culture is that relationships *are* important. This opposes the dominant culture, and thereby stokes up the dominant culture's antipathy towards the counter-culture. The therapy counter-culture can then express unflattering views about the scientific culture. Its scientificity may be dismissed as having no redeeming features, denigrated because it gives no room for the humanity of the patient. A somewhat unfair view that scientific psychiatry ignores the patient as a person leads the 'therapy culture' into difficult situations. It is not self-evident that psychotic patients always prefer a carer who emphasises the importance of relationships: in fact, the reverse. Schizophrenic patients prefer to remain isolated in their constructed world, and exert a control over others who would enter it (see Essay 2).

Proponents of the therapy culture will not always have the psychotic patient on their side.

Care, as simply relating humanely, is a rather sentimental view of the healing power of therapy. It lacks a toughness that has to be found in the standard psychiatric approach, which might nevertheless overplay that toughness in over-control. However, there is no doubt that psychotic patients, even the most institutionalised schizophrenic, can respond if the carer makes efforts to enter their world. But a connection with the patient is not necessarily therapeutic. As we saw in Essay 2 ('Understanding as a defence', p. 84), there is an important distinction between understanding and being understood. The analyst can gratify the patient by agreeing to *be* his self-understanding, and this links with the patients who require others to *be* their self-control, as we saw in Essay 1 ('Responsibility and professional identity', p. 12). This does not mean that efforts should not be made to engage, but we should be cautious as to when to claim therapeutic benefits. In fact, most carers who work in the therapeutic disciplines in psychiatry do not actually see psychotic patients for treatment. They tend to see patients with neurotic or personality disorders. Of course, there are exceptions: some psychoanalysts do make relations and conduct therapy with schizophrenic patients – Lucas (1993), Sohn (1999), Sinason (1993) for example in recent years. Most psychotherapists keep a distance from psychotic patients, though they use their own means, quite different from the dominant culture. Psychiatric doctors and nurses are physically present but preserve a degree of emotional distance, while psychotherapists are often physically removed. Psychotherapy is frequently conducted elsewhere in a separate department or clinic, with patients diagnosed with other conditions. Unfortunately, blinded by the retaliatory denigration expressed by the dominant scientific culture, the therapy culture overlooks how we are spared the really sharp end of the work. Often, psychotherapists offer themselves as consultants (or facilitators) for support groups for psychiatric teams, where they can encourage the staff to engage in closer relationships with schizophrenics: a practice that the therapist will not be advising for himself. In the extreme, psychotherapy services maintain a physical distance in units of their own, remote from the psychiatric service altogether. If the primary task is care of psychotic people, the therapy culture is almost totally dependent on the dominant culture for tackling that primary task directly, and on behalf of the whole institution.

It is important to be even-handed in understanding the mutual distortions arising from the contrasting motivations of separated subcultures. However, given that so often one of the subcultures is a dominant one, its distortions may seriously dominate the accomplishment of the task. To this end, it is important to address the particular and unexpected consequences of the distortion of the psychiatric service that arises from the 'scientific' attitudes, values and beliefs which have become dominant in psychiatry. One of the unacknowledged effects of the counter-culture is that its very existence in standing for 'human values', however distorted, has allowed the dominant culture to remain entrenched in its own complementary distortions.

Science

Psychiatry is an example of a culture with observable attitudes, including unspoken and unconscious ones. They have important effects on the perception and performance of the task. There are in the main two subsets of attitudes, two cultures: a dominant one and a counter-culture. The dominant one holds scientific attitudes that have some interesting properties. One interesting belief is that science does not have any 'attitudes'! The claim is that the quantification and generalisation inherent in doing science have eradicated human attitudes and values. Science believes it can claim to be neutral, and its results regarded as simply part of nature. Scientific facts are believed not to be reflected culturally through sets of attitudes or beliefs (see Rorty 1979). We are asked to conclude that scientific discoveries are simply facts of nature. This is philosophical realism – what you see is what you get. In fact, despite the success of technology, this argument has been under criticism since Kant and before. It is particularly limited in terms of the human sciences (see e.g. Bhaskar 1979). The notion that scientific facts are not influenced by personal or social beliefs is itself a belief.

Science as cultural attitudes

In practice we can observe implicit attitudes as to what is true, what is false and how to generate our evidence (Hinshelwood 2002). Scientific attitudes are particularly visible when people and their subjective experience are studied. As Main (1967) indicates in the quote given above (under 'Psychiatry and psychoanalysis', p. 124), from the point of view of natural science, people are systems of inanimate interactions. Such an inanimate object contrasts with persons having experiences. Patients are things that react, but in psychiatry we are asked to believe that they react as the inanimate things that science knows about. They react to drugs, ECT, cognitive instructions, etc. And we are asked to accept that people do not react to being the subject of scientific investigations. They only react within the parameters of the experiment and not to being the subject of the experiment. For instance, they are believed to react to the question 'How do you feel today?' only by stating how they feel. They are believed not to react to being questioned, to being the focus of attention, and so on.

This was Kraepelin's assertion, which was severely criticised by Laing (see 'The existential problem' in Essay 2, p. 73). It is an objective approach. Despite the handicap of depersonalising patients as inanimate things, for more than a century psychiatrists have made great headway in establishing objective criteria for the various psychiatric diagnoses, and for determining the quality and intensity of symptoms. Schneider's 'first rank symptoms' were a considerable advance 45 years ago in making the diagnosis of schizophrenia more reliable (Schneider 1959). The various depression scales allow one patient's affect to be compared more exactly with another's, or the comparison of one patient's state of mind at different times. These are important advances in making psychiatry objective. In the past 20 years the development of imaging machines has made progress in creating objective, visual images of states of mind. Psychology can be increasingly localised. The basic mental functions (and malfunctions) are being pinpointed in the material of the brain, and considerable relief has been afforded to suffering patients from this scientific approach. Considerable advances have been made possible by ignoring the experience of a subject being experimented with. Many patients have sufficient presence of mind to allow themselves without bother to be subjected to such objectification. Indeed, it is mostly the norm in general medicine to treat the body of the patient as a scientific object of study. Mostly patients agree to this and join the doctor and nurse willingly in thinking in an objective way about their bodies.

When the object of study is a patient's mind and his psychological experiences, the objective approach has a very different effect on the patient. If it is his actual person that is approached as his body might be, then he may react with discomfort and protest. If it is his person that requires attention, then an approach based on attitudes to the body can create profound difficulties. With psychotic patients these difficulties are very common. The schizophrenic person has a flaw in his sense of self anyway (see 'The existential problem' in Essay 2, p. 73), and as a result he experiences the investigations upon him in terms of his own problems. Frequently he fears them as bodily intrusions or depletions. In addition, scientific generalisations are depersonalising, and touch on his identity problems. In reaction, he may assume, in a very shallow way, all sorts of improbable identities.

As noted above, dominant attitudes in psychiatry view the object of study as a body rather than a person. If a person is one who asks that their world of experience be listened to, just as I think that we all do, the schizophrenic is disadvantaged because he already has a defective sense of being a person to whom we can listen. He hesitates to make that demand, and he is therefore particularly susceptible to a depersonalising attitude towards him. Doing science on him collaborates with his own self-depersonalisation (Hinshelwood 1999).

We now know that Schreber's father was a doctor who invented a method for the correct upbringing of children (Schreber 1903; Schatzman 1973; Shengold 1989). This imposed on the child a rigid military regime from early in life. Head braces, sleeping straps and exercises promoting ideal posture were recommended in the father's book (Schreber 1858). These ideas became widespread in Germany, in the nineteenth century, and Schreber Sr practised them upon his son. The Schreber family practised child care as a very mechanical process, placing this practice well in advance of human contact. They proclaimed correct posture rather than identity and meaning. A century later Harlow conducted experiments on Rhesus monkeys, rearing the young with figures made of wire to look like an adult monkey. The baby monkey could even suck this mechanical figure. The result, later in life, was a confusion about bonding to live monkeys (Harlow 1961). One cannot easily extrapolate from primates to humans with regard to schizophrenia (see however Bowlby 1969; Holmes 1993), but the schizophrenic's relatedness with the scientific professional is just as mechanical. Inserting the patient's head into an MRI scan, or some other physical and mechanical investigation, seems in this argument to be emblematic of the schizophrenic's loss of self and relationship with the external world. The patient is reduced to a world of interacting mechanical objects – to the patient's relief as well as the professionals', as we have seen. The purpose of such machinery is a good investigative one, but the relational context strikingly resembles the schizophrenic's depersonalised relations, and the Schreber scenario. So, despite the importance of the scientific approach to psychosis and the results on diagnosis and on outcome, there is a downside to it: a penalty for the patient and his treatment.

The schizophrenic's existential deficit may be aggravated by the objective process of investigation and treatment of his person. It is not that psychiatrists and psychiatric nurses do not make relationships with their patients: they do, simply by virtue of their own humanity. Not only that, but psychiatrists, nurses and most of us in the psychiatric service entered our careers because of a particular sympathy and interest in the pain of madness. Psychiatric staff are not uncaring, inhuman people; not at all. It is just that we have become in thrall to dominant attitudes in our profession, and that means we either create distance from the relationships through objective generalising attitudes (as in general psychiatry) or we sentimentalise them (as psychotherapeutically inspired staff may do). The genuine feelings for our patients remain, but remain silent. They have to be mediated through one or other set of given attitudes – dominant or counter-cultural attitudes.

What are the reasons for an allegiance to science? It would appear there are three separate ones. The first reason is that advances with great humanitarian benefit have resulted from the scientific approach. Second, there is a professional reason. Psychiatrists have an understandable ambition to be a respected profession. As a group, they wish to follow their medical colleagues, and that means seeking the accolades of scientific respectability.

Third, there is the much less visible force that concerns the psychology of being a psychiatric worker, which we have explored in Essay 1. A career as a psychiatric carer is usually entered into enthusiastically, but a daily caseload of suffering and disturbed persons quickly becomes draining work. It taxes the personal resources of psychiatric staff. In these circumstances, it is natural to create a distance from patients who arouse intense and continuous emotions that assault meaning and identity. The objectivity of a scientific approach demands emotional distance, a dispassionate objectivity. Therefore, the attitudes of science are ideal as a support for emotional *protection*. The more scientifically objective, the less emotionally vulnerable are the carers of disturbed people. The fit between the emotional neutrality of the scientific approach and the protective emotional distance is not unlike the fit between scientific attitudes and the schizophrenic's depersonalisation. Indeed, all three – the schizophrenic depersonalisation, the emotional protection of the staff, and the scientific attitude – go hand in hand. It is not surprising that scientific attitudes have become so robustly entrenched in the dominant set of attitudes and values in the culture of psychiatry.

Consequences of scientific beliefs

The scientific belief system, based on objectivity in attitude and neutrality of value, has become deeply rooted in Western culture over the past four centuries or so. Results of its technology have been enormous in terms of wealth and health. However, in turn it loops back to affect the way we see human beings, our own personal identity, and the nature of psychological disturbance. What is personal and relational drifts in the science lab to become a 'thing' as if it were almost physically real (see Weber 1954).

Reification

A good recent example of how human emotion is accommodated in the scientific mould is the concept of 'expressed emotion' in the family of the schizophrenic patient. The effects of a highly emotional family on the psychotic member are detrimental to the patient (Vaughn and Leff 1976). An objectifying attitude towards the relations of psychotic patients shows how implicitly the neutrality of a scientific approach 'reduces' a schizophrenic person's actual relations to a generalised concept. The quality of 'high expressed emotion' (HEE) can be objectified and quantified. The result is that this phenomenon, embedded in the experiences people have of each other, becomes a thing. It is reified. The quality of HEE becomes a measurable phenomenon in its own right. It loses connection with the persons from which it is emergent. In reality, there is no such thing as HEE separate from the people who express it, and receive it badly. Generalising it isolates and decontextualises the HEE entity in the interests of making it practically and clinically usable, but reifying this emotional interaction as a phenomenon in itself leaves the *persons* out of it. It becomes reconnected to the persons only through a statistical relation between the HEE score and the constellation of symptoms that constitute schizophrenia. It is not that personal relationships are overlooked *per se*; in fact, elucidating the HEE theory suggests sensitive initial observations on schizophrenics with their families. The point is that the attitudes that operate on this human sensitivity and awareness of the persons create an objectivity from which the persons inevitably fade.

It is important that this observation of the schizophrenic with her family has been made. However, once made it is 'reduced' to a statistical relation between the HEE score and a constellation of symptoms that is schizophrenia. There is nothing untoward about this, provided that this is all that happens. However, so often the statistical relationship begins to surmount and obliterate the personal relationship, in accordance with the injunction that personal relations are to be avoided. Then the empathy and sensitivity from which the original observation came shrink into the background. The objectified and impersonal (statistical) relationship supervenes.

This conversion from sensitivity to objectivity is useful in that it could point to personal relations between actual people. However, at the same time, it can be exploited unconsciously by researchers, carers and staff. It becomes that much harder to struggle back from objectivity to sensitivity; instead, a procedure based on the objective knowledge of HEE could be put into practice without anything more than a cursory acknowledgement of the actual participants under examination. So, the important lesson is to be aware of any retreat from personal relations to reified objects. To retain empathy with the suffering patient, and her family, there needs to be a binocular vision in which the pain and the statistics can be equally acknowledged.

Is it possible to 'do' science while also empathising with pain? The answer should be 'yes'. However, it is very understandable that in practice the answer is so often 'no'. Although the reasons for this are unconscious and supported by group pressures, there is no reason why the slippage from personal to statistical should not be acknowledged consciously, even if the detailed process cannot be. Of course, even better would be a willingness to enquire into the forces of the slippage from person to concept – and that is the *raison d'être* of this book. To proceed with the effects of the scientific approach and the implicit attitudes, I shall become rather abstract. I want to reach the abstract level of psychiatric research, which strengthens the implicit strategy of emotional distancing. Psychiatric research in the natural science mode of investigating inanimate things strongly supports the dominant mode of science in the clinical setting. One effect is to risk reducing options for treatment.

Treatment choices

Scientific attitudes towards the work – even the unspoken and unconscious attitudes – affect the patient's responses to treatment but, more than that, they can determine which treatments are on offer. Medical services assume that evidence for the profitable use of psychotherapy will flow from a scientific method. According to the UK Government agency NICE (National Institute for Clinical Excellence), there are five levels of scientific evidence – Types I–V. Type I, which is most valued, requires evidence from experiments conducted according to the drug-trial model known as the randomised control trial (RCT) method. Type II requires a variety of methods but one must be an RCT. Type III evidence is from controlled trials. Type IV comprises evidence from observational methods. And Type V, least valued, consists of the rest – clinical impressions, expert judgement, single-case studies, etc.

The highest standard for evaluating medical treatments, according to NICE, is the RCT, conducted with neither the subjects nor the researchers knowing the details (see Richardson 2001). This method emphasises a change in the symptoms and signs as the indicator of success for a treatment. Psychoanalytic psychotherapy has tended to rely on Type V evidence: clinical experience. Health providers in the public sector rely on scientific justification for economic expenditure, so the high-level Type I evidence is prioritised. Forms of evidence low down on the NICE list are no longer held to be a cogent evidence-base. As Holmes remarks:

> The drug treatment paradigm has enormous power in medicine. Research in psychological therapies, especially cognitive behaviour therapy, has been shaped by the 'drug metaphor'. (Holmes 2002, p. 290)

In other words, medical pressure asks us to regard a psychotherapeutic treatment as a drug treatment for purposes of research. The standard evidence is therefore the outcome study designed as an RCT, comparing one drug against another. Therefore one therapy must be compared against another therapy, a relevant drug, or placebo, any of which acts as the controlled variable. Holmes (2002) reviews five government and NHS publications on psychotherapy, and observes:

> In each of these publications due homage is paid to psychotherapy as a multifaceted, pluralistic enterprise in which a range of therapies is required to meet patient's various demands. Yet, when detailed recommendations are examined there is no doubt that cognitive behaviour therapy is promoted as the therapy of choice. (Holmes 2002, p. 288)

He concludes that this research discrepancy is so stark that 'Cognitive behaviour therapy is the therapy to beat' (p. 289). Roth and Fonagy (1996) also note the poor performance up to that time of outcome research in psychoanalysis and psychoanalytic psychotherapy. Cognitive behaviour therapy has reached this position because it has used the standard research format (the RCT) to report its effectiveness.

Certain psychotherapies, such as cognitive behavioural therapy (CBT), 'fit' the RCT, scientific model, while others do not. CBT relies on observing symptom change and in this account, CBT is taken as the paradigm of symptom change therapies. There is a fit between the demand for scientific evaluations and the cognitive conscious form of practice by CBT practitioners. Those which are relationship-based, such as psychoanalysis and psychoanalytic psychotherapy, have problems isolating variables that are usable in an RCT design. Therefore there is, simply, a lack of Type I evidence for psychoanalysis and psychoanalytic psychotherapy. A search of the Cochrane Library (a store of recent NICE-approved studies) revealed 48 abstracts for 'psychoanalysis' and 'psychoanalytic psychotherapy'; 'CBT' and 'cognitive behaviour therapy' produced 512. On this basis, scientific evidence for the benefit (or otherwise) of cognitive behaviour therapy is more than ten times that for, or against, psychodynamic therapies. These standards for research and research-led practice have been developing in the past decade, and have altered the availability of psychotherapies.

The poor harvest of RCT outcome studies of psychoanalytic psychotherapy treatments is sometimes regarded as reflecting a peculiar reluctance of psychoanalytic practitioners to submit their treatments to unbiased scrutiny. Practitioners are suspected of having something to hide – i.e. that their method doesn't work. Then, the supposed opposition by psychoanalytic psychotherapists to the new methods of outcome evidence is regarded as special pleading, a camouflage, and ultimately exploitation of patients. So, a renewed argument against psychoanalytic psychotherapy ensues.

Psychoanalytic psychotherapies, for their part, feel defensive, unnecessarily devalued, and that they are asked to jump through inappropriate hoops.[3] This sad interaction between practitioners of CBT and psychoanalytic psychotherapy is understandable, though regrettable. There may be some real validity in the described attitudes. Psychoanalytic psychotherapists may be particularly defensive; cognitive behaviour therapists may be devaluing of psychoanalysis. The point is that underlying the argument over RCT outcome studies, different assumptions are held by the opposing camps. It is a manifestation of the psychiatric schism.

In fact, at the time of writing, RCT-like trials of psychoanalytic psychotherapy are being planned, funded and conducted in increasing numbers – see for instance Emde and Fonagy (1997), Fonagy (1999) and Mace *et al.* (2000). Objectification and generalisation are quite possible in psychoanalytic research, as the thoughtful article by Hobson *et al.* (1998) indicates.

Research projects are under way for instance at Halliwick Day Hospital (Bateman and Fonagy 1999, 2001), at the Tavistock Clinic (Richardson 2001; McPherson *et al.* 2003) and at the Cassel Hospital (Chiesa and Fonagy 2000; Chiesa *et al.* 2002) in Britain. However, RCTs of psychoanalytic forms of treatment are difficult to plan and take much longer and thus are significantly more expensive, than those assessing other therapies. The design difficulties mean that the variables may be less precisely controlled and therefore results tend to be weakened to indications rather than proof. Leuzinger-Bohleber (2002) argued that different sciences of necessity have their own research methodology:

> Some leading philosophers of science (such as Hampe, 2000) state that this problem is not unique to psychoanalysis; all contemporary sciences have developed a research methodology specific to their subject and have developed their own criteria of scientific quality and 'truth'. (p. 3)

Persuading public funders to accept variable research methodologies may be very difficult. Fonagy remarks that 'It needs to be recognised

3 The correspondence in the *British Medical Journal* following Holmes (2002) http://bmj.com/cgi/eletters/324/7332/288_19176 and following) regretted in many cases the perceived opposition mentioned above and what is seen as special pleading on behalf of psychoanalytic psychotherapy.

that objections to research will not win the day' (Fonagy 2002, p. 58). Nevertheless, there is a risk of the range of therapies for needy patients being reduced. The principle advocated by Alanen *et al.* (1991) and other Scandinavian psychiatric services is to adapt the service to fit the patients' needs – the 'needs-adapted approach'. However, in services that are overly respectful of drug-trial research, as in the UK and the US, provision is coming to be tailored to 'scientific' outcome research rather than to patient need. This is true of an increasing number of countries as health costs have continuously risen. 'Managed care' policies align themselves with the same rationalist, realist, scientific principles.

However, psychiatry, in order to pursue its specific form of knowledge, needs to avoid following sheep-like the general medical trend until the debate has been properly argued.

Random controlled trials

Medical services assume almost exclusively that evidence for the profitable use of a treatment, including psychotherapy, will follow the standard medical drug-trial model. The standard form for medical outcome research, the RCT, was developed to compare drugs believed to be useful for a particular physical condition. In this experimental design, the experimenter varies the drug and this is known as the 'independent variable'. The experimenter then measures a change (if any) of an indicator (sign, symptom or test result) known as the 'dependent variable'. The RCT method was developed to exclude all variables other than the drug treatment and the indicator of change. The method was designed and adopted to exclude subjective psychological factors such as suggestion, the 'bedside manner' and the placebo effect. The key requirement is the objective indicator of change – usually a change in pathological signs (such as blood levels of specific substances, bodily lumps etc., or physiological functions). The model experiment objectively compares two or more treatments on the basis of their impact on the same specific indicator. Usually a new drug treatment is compared on the same indicator with an old or accepted treatment. Therefore the aim is to compare like with like. Crucial to this is an objective quantification of the independent and dependent variables.

In psychiatry, objectification is problematic in a way that it is not in physical medicine. The role of objective pathological test results is minimal, therefore change is inevitably based on the subjective experience of the patient or the staff. Psychiatric research in the past half-century made good headway in rendering subjective reporting by patients into more objectively sound and quantitative measures. That objectification usually requires careful questionnaire or interview techniques, with large populations of patients, processed by sophisticated statistical methods (see for instance Guntrip (1967)). This is an important research strategy, but it is less useful in the clinical situation with individual patients. In clinical practice, change is actually gauged by subjective criteria, which cannot be reduced to statistical data.

The strength of CBT is that it can be made objective in this way. Serial questionnaire ratings of frequency and intensity of symptoms resemble the indicators used in drug-trial research, and reduce the element of subjectivity. CBT resembles the standard model of medical evidence, the RCT, because of the measured symptom change it uses. However, evidence based on symptom change in CBT only allows a comparison with other therapies that assess symptom change. In practice, not all therapies rely on symptom change as the dependent variable. Psychoanalytic treatment is the paradigm therapy that aims more than anything at *relationship change.*

Relational therapies

Unfortunately, relationship changes are more difficult to reduce to objective assessment. Relations may be indicated by symptom change, but the two kinds of change are not reliably correlated. This is particularly stark with certain patients whose presenting problem is a relational one, and not an explicit symptom. In fact, this group of borderline and other personality disorders is currently the main field of operation for psychoanalysis and psychoanalytic psychotherapy.

So, comparison between symptom-based and relationship-based therapies is unsatisfactory because there is no common indicator to allow a valid like-with-like comparison. If change is assessed in terms of a single indicator (the symptom), we reduce the field to a single treatment (CBT) that is not comparable with others. But if change is conceived in terms of different outcome indicators – symptom change for one treatment and relation change for another – then no true comparison of therapy with therapy can occur. The demands of clinical governance for valid comparison cannot be satisfied. The RCT design needs a single indicator, and it has not got one in psychotherapy. So, the RCT is very restricted as an instrument to compare symptom-change therapies and relationship-based therapies.

Placebo or transference

The RCT was designed specifically to evaluate the physical, bodily effects of drugs. Very specifically it aimed to control – and thus exclude – the effects and biases that come from emotional attitudes towards treatment (hope, fear, etc.). It also excludes, by intention, the effects of reassurance, suggestion and the placebo effect. These usual effects of the care relationship are suspect because they are extraneous to the knowledge required. The RCT was designed specifically to rule out relationship effects of treatments. The RCT design is predicated on a realist set of assumptions – i.e. there is a fact to be found which transcends all personal or social attitudes or influences.

The placebo effect is exactly what the drug trial does not want to interfere in the treatment, yet a relational psychotherapy exploits precisely that 'placebo effect'. The 'treatment alliance' and 'transference' are the essential and focal elements of psychoanalysis. They are quintessentially relationships, subjective and a mutual influence on subject and experimenter. We can seriously question whether the RCT method, which was developed precisely to eliminate the placebo effect, is appropriate for assessing a method based on the treatment relationship as the indicator of outcome.

Moreover, psychoanalysis takes a neutral stance on whether the transference (or placebo effect) is positive or negative, while CBT is particularly dependent on compliance – the CBT method wins the patient's co-operation and is ineffective in non-compliant patients. Psychoanalysis is in a sense 'compliance-neutral', focusing specifically on the care relationship, whether compliant or non-compliant. In fact, it could be said that analysing transference is a treatment focused on the nature and extent of compliance itself. Because of that, it could even be argued, with some irony, that psychoanalysis is more in line with the spirit of the RCT method than a compliance-dependent treatment.

More tellingly still, the emotional neutrality of the RCT is itself beginning to come under suspicion. There is now a concern that in trials funded by drug companies, their commercial interest will be reflected in the gratitude of the researchers, who will unwittingly seek results so as not to disappoint their funders. Curiously, there is no longer a complete confidence that RCTs can counter this. Elaborate disclosure of interests is increasingly required in reported research.

Social construction

Another dimension to the problem of scientific objectivity in psychiatry (and even in medicine) is the effect of social pressures on the subjectivity that we study and try to convert into objective phenomena. Social factors create serious issues for objective methods in psychotherapy. Symptoms and their derivatives, syndromes, are socially constructed in many cases (Figlio 1982). Socially expected categories of ill-health, together with a negotiation between the patient and doctor (or therapist), can 'construct' a diagnosis. In general medicine, there is usually a fail-safe mechanism in biological testing through objective physiological and anatomical findings. But no similar fail-safe exists for problems of the mind. Social construction challenges the view that objective phenomena transcend social and personal attitudes. It suggests that these apparently objective phenomena depend on human attitudes, values and relations. For example, the massive excess of schizophrenic diagnoses in Afro-Caribbean members of the British population, as well as the disproportionate use of medication, implies that psychiatry operates with stereotyped views of certain immigrant groups. Such attitudes massively affect diagnosis, however objective the criteria. Objective methods in psychiatry cannot realistically ignore the relational framework of social attitudes subjectively held.

The psychiatric drive to objectify symptoms and diagnoses takes place inevitably in a framework made up of social attitudes held by doctors, patients and society at large. Psychiatric diagnoses are therefore particularly prone to 'fashion' in different historical periods, when symptoms and syndromes can be 'constructed' socially. One instance is the peak of interest in, and diagnosis of, multiple personality disorder in the 1890s and again in the 1990s. Such a diagnosis retreated largely into oblivion in the intervening period. Inevitably, we would have to look for social and cultural reasons for the peaks and troughs in that historical story.

If psychiatric symptoms, syndromes and diagnoses are in part (a greater or lesser part) socially constructed by the common attitudes among patients and doctors, then 'cures' are just as likely to be socially constructed from the same ingredients – social expectations and the care relationship. A cure based on such 'subjective' ingredients is no less a cure, and indeed objectifying such changes may be possible. However, we need to be aware that social attitudes to medicine, to psychiatry and to human nature itself underpin the objective criteria just as much as scientific facts do.

Scientific management

One of the interesting things about this cultural movement within psychiatry towards scientific attitudes is that a similar movement, occurring outside psychiatry, has a bearing on our service. A new management culture has come into the British NHS over the past two decades or so, and has come into the healthcare culture of other societies a little later. In Britain, ever since the 1973 National Health Service Re-organisation Act, changes have involved more integrated management and local accountability, and the generation of a national 'evidence-base' for the choice of treatments. It is a style of management known as 'scientific management' (Taylor 1911), and it respects the rational basis of the organisation's work and the rational attitudes with which all members of the organisation approach their work. It keys in closely with the same increasingly scientific attitudes in the practice of psychiatry.

In 1983 the 'Griffiths report' recommended the introduction of general management into the NHS as it had become standard in other industries (Griffiths 1983). Continual further discussion led to the introduction of the 'internal market' in 1991, with the enormous increase in financial control and competition, and an enhanced demand for accountability of money spent from the public purse. General management methods and systems were greatly enhanced to cope with the competitive and accountability requirements that had to be met by local trading units, called 'NHS Trusts'. By 1999, the emphasis had changed from market competition and central financial accountability to stressing the scientific credentials of treatments offered. The National Institute for Clinical Excellence (NICE) was established then. It was charged to ensure the provision of 'authoritative, robust and reliable guidance on current "best practice" '. That change was to gauge best practice as the best proven treatments, and no longer (as before 1999) the best market performers. The question arose of how to find the best practice, and evidence for this is now enshrined in audits undertaken by NICE. The Cochrane Library also continuously surveys research results that pertain to the effectiveness of treatments. National Service Frameworks (NSFs) are documents that review standards of treatment in a particular speciality or for a particular condition, and establish the evidence base for treatments.

For 20 years, this new business culture has been continuously introduced and strengthened. New rational management systems have sharply increased as the required method of delivery of medical care, and this is driven by health costs as they have reached a ceiling that demands a system of rationing. This is a world-wide phenomenon, but in Britain, at least, the culture of management has painfully impinged on the culture of care. Interestingly, this pair of pre-existing sets of attitudes – management and clinical cultures – have come together within the NHS and formed a cultural schism that has a similar pattern to others described in this essay (see 'Schisms', p. 119). The care culture is committed to care for the ailing; management culture is survival of the fittest with the ailing being pushed over the cliff. Adjusting to the painful, poignant conflict implicit in health rationing, the two cultures have polarised into distorted attitudes that oppose each other.

1 The care culture embodies the attitude that the sick need help and support to recover. With this attitude, cost problems are dismissed. There is a blithe disregard for resource limits. Attitudes to money simply mean demands for more of it. Clinicians cause a considerable frustration among the managers who react to this apparent irresponsibility.
2 The management culture embodies the attitude that competition and survival depend on efficient and healthy functioning. Managers cause clinicians dismay at apparently inhumane arguments and decisions.

This clash has driven the two sides apart, leaving many carers struggling to reconcile conflicting and distorted attitudes. Care loses a sense of reality, and management loses a capacity for leadership. Both are reduced, but the distortions offer some relief to both sides. They help both to avoid the pain of rationing: clinicians demand more resources and feel on the side of the angels, while managers keep their heads in their accounts and avoid seeing the impact of cuts.

Instead of a long, hard look at this uncomfortable reality, there is a clash of attitudes. They seem oppositional and have driven the two sides into polarities. Once again an escape from a nasty conflict is externalised as a conflict between groups, between managers and clinicians. At the same time as this incipient schism between managers and clinicians proceeds, within medicine another process is occurring. Scientific management promotes assumptions that are also held by the dominant mode in psychiatry. The newer scientific management can be a potent support for the particular dominant attitudes in psychiatry. An alliance with scientific management promises psychiatry greater influence. It can strengthen the view that only human rationality should exist at work, and emotional attitudes and distress can be eradicated.

Reactions to the scientific culture

The counter-culture in psychiatry resists the obliterating quality of the scientific attitude in psychiatry. But there have been two cogent reactions on a broader scale – one against the single-minded enthusiasm for evidence-based practice in medicine, and one against the broader scientific management culture.

Narrative-based practice

Psychiatry has followed the medical trend in establishing an objective evidence-base, deriving from the RCT research design. However, we risk doing violence to the delicate subjectivity of our kind of study, which Wallerstein characterised as 'the quintessentially mental concerns of desire and will and intention in all their subjectivity and elusiveness and ambiguity that are, indeed, the essence of psychoanalysis' (Wallerstein 2000, p. 39). It is therefore of considerable interest to psychoanalysts that within the movement for evidence-based medicine, similar doubts have surfaced that there is a risk of something being lost.

> The conventional case history . . . represents, at best, the intersection between a particular patient world and the abstract world of medical knowledge, about which patients may know little. The core clinical skills of listening, questioning, delineating, marshalling, explaining and interpreting provide a potential mediation between these different worlds. Yet as Michael Balint

> pointed out, whether these tasks are performed well or badly is likely to have as much influence on the outcome of the illness from the patient's point of view as the more scientific and technical aspects of diagnosis or treatment. (Greenhalgh and Hurwitz 1998, pp. 13–14)

Balint's work, at one time a widespread movement especially in general practice, emphasised the importance of the personal relationship in care (Balint 1957). According to these views, the something that is missing is narrative. '[N]arrative is absorbing. It engages the listener and invites an interpretation' (Greenhalgh and Hurwitz 1998, pp. 3–4). Narratives offer meaning, context and perspective, and 'encourage empathy and promote understanding between clinician and patient' (p. 7), all of which are normally bleached from evidence gained by methods of objectification. This plea for the place of narrative in the practice of medicine is the more remarkable for the fact that Greenhalgh is Director of a unit for evidence-based practice, where she teaches and researches evidence-based practice. Turning to narrative indicates that the evidence-based movement is attempting to reach a more balanced view of practice. Narrative is the way in which the subject can be reinstated into the clinical encounter:

> In acknowledging the interpretive nature of clinical understanding, we are forced to reject the notion of pure objectivity, for the very existence of interpretive possibilities implies subjectivity, ambiguity and room for disagreement. (Greenhalgh 1998, p. 257)

In this vein, Anna Donald (1998) presses even further in trying to redress the balance. She describes the very change from medical expert to evidence-based medicine as itself a narrative, observing that the death of the expert as truth-giver espoused in evidence-based management is reminiscent of the denouncement of priestly experts that took place during the Reformation (pp. 24–25). She draws on Ian Hacking's account of modern science as an interpretative narrative (Hacking 1999). That narrative of the displaced expert, like the scientific narrative, is not necessarily endorsed by patients (Hacking 1999, Kleinman 1988).

Robert Platt found himself shocked, after a lifetime of teaching medical students, by the unnatural emphasis on generalisations in medical education:

> The first staggering fact about medical education is that after two and a half years of being taught on the assumption that everyone is the same, the student has to find out for himself that everyone is different, which is what his experience has taught him since infancy. (Platt 1965, p. 551)

This plea is echoed by Howard Brody in his foreword to Greenhalgh and Hurwitz (1998): 'Some of medicine works extremely well precisely because it treats people as all being the same; and some of medicine works very well because it treats people as different' (p. xiii). Brody argues emphatically that narrative 'connects the teller and the listener' (p. xiii), i.e. the patient with the doctor. The conclusion is that we must restore relationships to the practice of medicine, from which relational effects have been bleached by the use of scientific rationality. Such a reaction to scientific medicine and psychiatry always risks sounding like a battle-cry. A measured tone is most appropriate, to engage in a rapprochement. To complement the aims of 'narrative-based practice', we must understand why the divorce of evidence from narrative took place and has endured so tenaciously. If those forces are not reckoned with, there will be no rapprochement.

Emotional labour

Similarly, a second reaction to scientific management echoes the narrative-based movement. Its critique of scientific management rediscovers emotions, and the fact that people take them to work. It reinstates a serious study of emotion at work. Emotions play a significant part in healthcare as well as rationality. Hochschild (1983) first formulated clearly the fact that workers in the service industries must labour on their own emotional states (see also Fineman 1993; Linstead and Hopfl 2000). They are required, as part of employment, to produce the correct emotional response (e.g. a smile) whatever the service user is like, and whatever the relationship between provider and user. Flight attendants in the airline industry are expected (and even trained) to have the emotional responses that will benefit the company. They are required, *as company policy*, to smile even when abused (!) and to abolish anger from their display. There is regular training to this effect. The bedside manner of doctors and nurses is a similar example of the way service workers, including professional carers, have to work on their emotional reactions. Emotional labouring demands a management of the self, and implies that emotions can be brought under control of rationality in an unproblematic way. However, Hochschild has also stressed that there has to be a sincerity, a degree of conviction in the display of the required emotion. What is demanded is not a mere formula of words, a nonchalant 'have a nice day' gesture. The job done by actors in a theatre is somewhat similar. Whatever their actual state, they are required, Paggliacci-like, to produce the correct emotional performance. It is a performance of emotional states so evident that it should move an audience. This requires some clear separation of their actual emotional state from a capacity to know another one, and to display it with convincing depth.

A nurse must convey some real interest in the person, and in his pain and dread. The assumption of this approach is that this kind of work can be consciously contrived to a high level of conviction. In fact, surprisingly, this can be achieved. The best actors, for instance, can project a required emotional experience to the back of the gallery. The capacity to achieve this kind of emotional work means that the mind is capable of separating into different parts:

(a) one that can internally observe what is going on,
(b) two parts, at least, that can be occupied by the different emotional states (for example the anger and the smile),
(c) a repository of latent emotional states which can act as an inventory from which to select the required display,
(d) a system for choosing between emotional states, and
(e) some motivation to operate this system.

Hopfl and Linstead (1993) have also noted this multiplicity of 'selves'. It requires a complex psychology to explain this phenomenon. The psychoanalytic paradigm can certainly contribute something about the division of the self and how those parts interact, but this is a large project which involves a contribution of psychoanalysis to the sociology of emotion (Clarke 2003; Craib 1998).

Within the rationalist framework of scientific management, the motivating principle is assumed to be monetary earnings. However, it is striking that often those who have the most arduous of emotional labour to perform are the least well paid. Those nurses most closely attending sick, frightened or dying patients are notoriously badly paid compared with senior staff who sustain a greater distance.

This would imply motivations other than money. Psychoanalysis points towards unconscious motives connected with human concern for others. This is a universal human response, probably biologically supported to allow the evolution of socialisation. It involves deep psychological layers, as we have seen in Essay 1 (p. 21). Concern for a drunken passenger in the plane can lead to a modification of the flight attendant's anger with him when he swears at her. This angle on concern in the work is invariably overlooked. At least, it is overlooked *as work*. Instead, it is regarded as a competence for which simple training is all that need be provided, and without recognition that emotional work demands deep clefts in the experience the person has of herself. There is also concern in the flight attendant for the airline company, which is an object that needs care. The company presents itself as dependent on its employees and on their willingness to support its policy.

Risks and rituals

As Theodosius concluded from her study of emotions in nursing practice, agency for patient and nurse is derived from *both* rational and emotional sources (Theodosius 2003). If this is true of general medicine, it must be enormously more true of psychiatry, where the irrational and the emotional are the very field of study and interaction. In the psychiatric service, there is a need for staff to preserve a professional calm while confronting madness and violence, with all the fears that such confrontation evokes. Irma Brenman-Pick says something similar about the psychoanalyst's work, which creates a similar 'ambiguous problem, this walking the tightrope between experiencing disturbance and responding with interpretation that does not convey disturbing anxiety' (Brenman-Pick 1985, p. 157). This is a critical event that a psychiatric carer has to live through all day, every shift. It is a process that demands an extreme distortion and cleavage in the self, a psychological contortion. Generally psychiatric workers understand this impact on themselves, and accept it – not for monetary gain particularly, but because of the motivations described in Essay 1. However, the onslaught is sufficiently intense, and sufficiently neglected, for psychiatric workers to find themselves distinctly disabled by the experiences, and the impact and cleavage in themselves takes on a different scale from that of airline flight attendants.

The management of emotion, which is promoted by a 'scientific' management, has its basis in rational views of the work and, by extension, of the emotions appropriate for the work. In such a rationalist philosophy, these appropriate emotions can simply be assumed by the worker in an unproblematic way. They are in a sense reasonable emotions to have. Management discourse excludes the irrational. Since, for better or worse, the irrational is a part of human beings, it moves into a twilight zone underground, or unconscious. The consequence of such 'denial' is that inevitably it must become unmanageable.

Regrettably, only the marginal points of view, such as a psychoanalytic one, can fully acknowledge the existence and even the effects of those unspoken emotional currents. Painful emotional states, or anxiety, are not entirely overlooked, but instead rational solutions are applied in ways that continue to depersonalise the experience at this underground level. Not only psychiatric staff react to the impact of psychosis. Families, relatives, friends and neighbours are affected in the same way. The authorities responsible for healthcare and for law and order also become suffused with anxieties and concern about control of madness; they *become* the self-control. Indeed, anxiety about madness is rife. It percolates up to government and, at the same time, a control function percolates up. The self-control of the patient migrates through the social relations – from relatives, to the professional psychiatric service, to higher management, the public media and to government. There are therefore concerns all the way up through responsible officials and elected politicians, resulting in ever more centralised control. Layers of controllers controlling the 'controllers' gradually emerge in, and evoke, a bureaucracy. This means progressive alienation of the initiative and decision-making of increasing numbers of professionals, managers and politicians, and not just of patients. As anxieties ascend the escalator of social hierarchy more procedures are put in place, so that people follow them rather than their own agency.

The buck that is passed is in a psychoanalytic sense a particle of the patient's alarm at his own potential loss of control and coherence (as in the example near the beginning of this essay of the man asking not to be let out of prison, on p. 112). The particle of emotion transforms and amplifies (Hinshelwood 1989a, 2001) in its journey through various roles and persons, and in its course invariably loses its personal quality. The alienated particle then embarks on a career as a generalised issue of public concern. Finally, it returns as a set of procedures that professionals shall observe. This career for an abandoned part of a person is not unusual (Hinshelwood 1989a, 1989b), but it is particularly common and particularly forceful when we consider psychotic fragmentation and dispersal. Something, once personal and impulsive, has become generalised, impersonal, routinised and alienated. Because of the requirement for meticulous observance of procedures, any risk-management protocols can be followed 'mindlessly', and the professional comes to deal with her patients in as depersonalised a way as psychotic patients feel about themselves.

More and more centralised efforts to think about 'risk' and to design methods of 'risk management' are now the accepted way of dealing with anxieties.[4] Dull monotonous, predictable regularity is a common strategy for control in the psychiatric services (other institutions, such as prisons, have similar strategies). At the very least, a strict predictability is designed to eradicate the unpredictability of incoherent psychosis. Dull predictability is mind-numbing, and is intended to lull the potentially psychotic mind into insensibility. It is understandable as a strategy in an anxious institution. However, the serious side-effect is the alienation of personal relations and careful thought.

Main (1967) plotted the course in a small institution by which the loss of thought happened. He described how, in a therapeutic community, procedures are developed by a flexible approach to the real problems that crop up all the time when people are living together. Such reality-based solutions to problems are then handed on from one generation to another. They change, however, in this intergenerational passage. They become 'the way things are done' – they ossify and become rigid and unthinking. Memories of why they are done this way are forgotten, often quickly, and a moral tone takes over from the original practical one. In psychoanalytic terms, Main says that the particular procedure changes its residence from the ego to the super-ego, from problem-solving to a quasi-religious injunction. It stops being a realistic solution to become an (often enforced) unthinking ritual. On a societal scale, the manualisation of procedures, and even an aspect of evidence-based medical practice, is a similar strategy to institutionalise an 'ought' injunction, in place of

4 Risk-management applies only to the conscious element of anxiety. Unconscious anxieties about the work and about performance and achievement remain inevitably unattended by a rationalist approach. They are managed unconsciously according to all the methods described in Essay 1 and this essay.

an authentic problem-solving struggle.[5] The depleting of initiative involved in this strategy goes against the attempts to restore human potential and personhood to people who have given them up.

Risk-management protocols and ritualised manuals contain an extraordinary amount of wisdom. Yet they preserve it in a form that can be deadening. Much of the well-meaning attempt to take over the self-control and the self-knowledge of psychotic patients has led to maladaptive interpersonal phenomena, and ultimately to organisational processes in which the individual, whether patient or staff, becomes alienated from herself.

Alienation

There is no *conscious* working at the emotional labour that is demanded of psychiatric carers. The psychiatric worker slides into a set of attitudes that replace the emotional labour with an unthinking emotional distance. This is then supported by the demands of the scientific culture of psychiatric units and by the patients themselves, who so often wish intently to turn away from the reality of their feelings and their relationships. In addition, that distancing is supported by the 'scientific' management that concentrates on the rationality of the workers. The neglect, the lack of empathy in the system and the forcing down of financial reward demoralise the worker further. She becomes a person who is divided in herself without recognition. That self-alienation approaches the existential predicament of the schizophrenic patient.

We have described the nature of institutionalisation as an enduring system in which parts of the identity of the self are redistributed such that all staff are healthy and wise, all patients helpless and grateful. Patients lose their agency, which is to be re-found in the enhanced sense of power within the staff (see Essay 1, 'Responsibility and professional identity', p. 12). Denis Martin described institutionalisation in the large and traditional mental hospital:

> the patient has ceased to rebel against, or to question the fitness of his position in a mental hospital; he has made a more or less

5 Main concluded that the way to cope with this potentially lethal process is to sustain a process of thinking about 'the way things are done'. Continually asking 'What is the problem that this is a solution to?' then respects reality, restores initiative and, interestingly, sustains a culture of enquiry (Main 1967; Norton 1992; Griffiths and Hinshelwood 1997).

> total surrender to the institution's life . . . he is co-operative. Here 'co-operative' usually implies that the patient does as he is told with a minimum of questioning or opposition. This response on the part of the patient is very different from that true co-operation essential to the success of any treatment, in which the patient strives to understand, and work with, the doctor in his efforts to cure . . . [The] patient, resigned and co-operative . . . too passive to present any problem of management, has in the process of necessity lost much of his individuality and initiative. (Martin 1955, pp. 1188–1190)

The patient has lost his power and agency. He has lost individuality, initiative, enquiry and self-determination. He has lost his active self. This is a gross state of self-alienation. His identity has been depleted of an essential aspect of himself. More than that, it stands apart from him, actually in the form of a member of staff – or, more accurately, in the identity of a member of staff.[6] As we saw in Essay 1, the distortion of identity in terms of professional responsibility and self-responsibility ultimately affects the staff as well as the patient, and in turn that 'buck' of responsibility moves ever upwards, leaving those lower down in a state depleted of initiative and agency. Entrance into that old-fashioned psychiatric institution was an entrance into a psychological system in which the patient became alienated from a large part of himself through fundamental splitting mechanisms, which distorted and mutilated his identity.

There is a kind of relocation of healthy individuality. Staff get more of it; patients lose what they have left of it. There is a kind of redistribution of health. But this occurs at the next step up the hierarchy too. This is a system that distributes active and responsible parts of the person. There are links to be seen with the wider economic and social system, and the similarly unequal distribution of wealth. It may look far-fetched to link an economic system of distribution with a psychological one, but the parallels seem so remarkable that we need to consider them seriously. Psychoanalytic descriptions of the depleted states when splitting and projection take place can be shown to resemble Marx's description of alienation in mid-nineteenth century workers (Hinshelwood 1983). For instance, 'The worker becomes poorer the more wealth he produces, the more

6 Such disruptions of the supposedly indivisible individual are dealt with elsewhere (Hinshelwood 1997).

his production increases in power and extent' (Marx 1844, p. 323). In these *1844 Economic and Philosophical Manuscripts*, alienation is described as a depleted psychological state: 'the object that labour produces, its product, stands opposed to it as something alien, as a power independent of the producer' (Marx 1844, p. 324). He talks of a kind of 'objectification' of the work. The worker loses the product of his skills and creativity, in the act of appropriation of his production by others. He becomes estranged from something that was his own power and creative work. The object 'stands opposed', as Marx says, *alien* and *independent*, having absorbed something of the worker. In other words, products of the person's (worker's) body are felt to have become separated off, to become located as a characteristic of someone else: 'the more powerful the alien, objective world becomes which he brings into being over and against himself, the poorer he and his inner world become and the less they belong to him' (p. 324). This is a very precise description which could be just as accurate about the process a psychiatric patient is involved in, by which his own self-governance and initiative come to 'stand opposed' to him, alien and independent in the form of his psychiatric carers. In these processes, which psychoanalysts call splitting and projection, one person is psychologically depleted while others become built up. So, Marx described the relocation of personality characteristics in a strikingly similar way to the relocation of wealth.

Marx's early attempt to understand the psychological plight of the worker in the exploitative industrial system parallels remarkably the psychological description made a century later by psychoanalysts working with psychotic patients. There is therefore a significant correspondence between the expropriation of a worker's physical labour and material production, and the expropriation of a psychotic patient's being. The possibility exists that in a social system such as that which has grown up in Western society, there is a particular form of alienation of individuals which detaches them from themselves, or from significant parts of themselves: their power or their labour (Hinshelwood 2000). Psychoanalytically, this is splitting and projection; socially, this is alienation. Moreover, we can consider whether our culture particularly prompts exploitation in these various areas of social relations.

This argument has meandered into wider social forms of alienation which form the social context. The serious point to conclude on is that the psychiatric worker in community care is not spared the impact of any of the processes that beset the carer in a large old-fashioned institution. The newer institutions in community care – the hostels, day centres and hospitals, the in-patient wards and all the agencies we now use – are in the firing line of the impact of psychosis, and can no less develop institutional pathology which can distort identity, confuse meaning, and lead to task drift and to schism within the service. This does not have to be a gloomy conclusion so long as we learn these lessons, and are ready to spot the problems that arise through processes invisible to the rationalist approach.

Epilogue

Being psychotic, being a person

When we considered Conran's description of an admission to a mental hospital, we summarised the process of projection into the hospital staff (Essay 1, 'Responsibility and professional identity', p. 12). In that paper, interestingly, Conran compared the psychotic's admission with that of a quite normal person admitted as an emergency to a surgical ward with acute appendicitis. In the latter case too, Conran described a process whereby the patient in pain and feeling extremely unwell gave up his own initiative and agency. His capacity for self-care was lost as he took himself to bed and asked his wife to call the doctor. In subsequent steps, his self-care was passed to the wife, then the doctor, and then the hospital and the surgeon. Finally, as he recovered after the operation, his body healed and the split in his personality also healed. He could 'take back these projected parts of himself, resume the government of himself and take his discharge' (Conran 1985, p. 35): a fluent process of splitting and projective identification, followed by a return of the projected parts and restoration of his initiative and agency for himself. The processes that we have seen as fundamental to the psychotic condition – splitting and projective identification – are therefore to be seen as occurring in quite significant and painful form in the ordinary person. This patient too became alienated from himself for a while.

Conran's comparison leads us to consider the difference between the psychotic and the normal person when they embark on a process of splitting and projective identification. As we saw in Essay 1 (p. 18), the alienation of the psychotic patient did not reverse to a restoration of the person. Two years after she left hospital, the woman was still demanding in a powerful and uncomfortable way that the doctor do her knowing for her. He had still to *be* her self-knowledge. This was quite different from the ordinary surgical patient, for whom the restoration of the psychological splitting flowed smoothly from the healing of the surgical wound.

The smooth cycle was interrupted in the case of the schizophrenic patient. She retained the psychological condition in which her projected self was embodied by the hospital and the doctor. A pathological *status quo* endured for years. What prompted that psychological stasis within the relationship? Consequently, to what extent can an understanding of that factor contribute to a specific strategy for relating to psychotic patients?

Something got stuck in the hospital and staff, in Conran's example. It was the capacity to know. Or rather, it was specifically the experience of not knowing: of feeling something meaningless, something that could not be understood, or could only be known as something that could not be made sense of. Conran called it 'nameless dread' (after Bion 1962a). It would appear that precisely this projective system is the cause of trouble for the treatment of schizophrenia. The problem therefore seems to be compounded of a number of factors:

- a stuck projective system; the alienation of initiative in one group, the patients;
- the projection of something which, for want of a better expression, is the transfer of meaninglessness;
- the creation of institutions that can harbour these occurrences where their existence has to be denied in favour of reasonable emotion;
- a wider social culture that enhances a quality of alienation or depersonalisation in each of these factors.

If we bring these factors together, from many points in the course of the three essays, we complete the landscape that arises in our service from the impact of psychosis. Similarly, we can bring together certain hints about what might be employed to mitigate these effects. It is important to recognise at the outset that work with actual patients is not going to address any factors arising from the wider culture. Deleuze and Guatari (1972), critiqued psychoanalysis, probably correctly, for ignoring these wider social effects of the exploitative alienating and depersonalising effects of the culture we live within (see also Holland 1999). Having acknowledged this, we can then ask how the psychiatric carer can develop a practice that can mitigate those factors that are within the realm of the psychiatric services.

Sections in Essay 1 (pp. 43–46) deal with internal and external consultancy and the special requirements for that function in working with psychotics. The capacity for reflection has been closed off in the schizophrenic patient and, with powerful force, any reflective space in the psychiatric team or in the individual staff also comes under pressure. Limited thought means more opportunity to enact roles such as the forensic patient ('Unconsious interpersonal systems' in this essay, p. 111), and indeed the creation of patient and staff stereotypes (Essay 1, 'Institutionalisation', p. 13). Thoughtful reflection is necessary on the possible ways in which staff find themselves acting in the work, and is also a powerful means of capturing some sense of the schizophrenic's distress.

Reflection, derived from external or internal consultancy, creates understanding. As we saw in Essay 1 ('Action and understanding', p. 20), understanding may be of various kinds: (a) listening into the experience that is being expressed by another person; (b) professional understanding in the form of a diagnosis; (c) the odd non-symbolic method of communicating through action on another person's mind. In Essay 2 we added a further detail. There is the potential for a defensive kind of understanding, in which an easy explanation is offered and gratefully received (see p. 85). That explanation evades the full pain of the psychotic experience for both parties. The pain has a particular relation to knowledge and understanding. In less severe disturbance, psychoanalysis postulates a conflict between wishes – between sex and survival, or between life and harm. However, in the more severe disturbances, the problem appears to be much more to do with the impossibility of understanding. When Conran was confounded by the phone call to his ex-patient of three years, he was aghast as she emphasised her incomprehension. She did it in a way that filled him with just the same painful feeling of incomprehension. Thus, psychosis appears to involve a trade in meaninglessness. Therefore it is tempting to find meanings that preempt that painful meaninglessness. We saw just that dynamic interplay in Essay 2, when the analyst Murray Jackson interviewed Anthony, a schizophrenic with a compulsion to burn himself (p. 94). It appeared that Anthony could not bear the interviewer to suggest meaningful links with his hallucinations and delusions, but was much more responsive when the interviewer began to ask questions from a position of not knowing (see p. 96). Then Anthony seemed able to ally himself with help, but only when he found another mind capable of not-knowing, and thus capable of tolerating a sense of not having a meaning. At the point where he felt the interviewer coming with him into meaninglessness, he could even begin to move towards the awfulness of the actual meaning that blew his mind apart.

Although the meaninglessness of a schizophrenic patient seems to warrant turning away from him in futility, there is a point to listening to his meaninglessness; the point is that he may be able to join you in the futility, when meanings are beyond him. From that point of feeling that his meaninglessness is understood, there are new possibilities. It is a support sufficient in some cases to move towards the intolerable meaning. The upshot of this is that reflection on the work may have to start with a recognition of not-knowing. It may be rather like the frustrating experience of the worker in the example of the schism (Essay 3, 'Psychiatry and psychoanalysis', p. 124), who recognised the need for 'not-doing' and, moreover, the need for a space to reflect on that not-doing.

It appears to be a paradoxical situation if we, as professional experts, exist in a state of not-knowing (or not-doing). As professionals, we are expected to know things and what to do about them. However, our expertise in psychosis is precisely about not-knowing, and the toll that it takes on the mental health of both patient and staff.

There are a number of features of the reflection needed in working with psychosis:

- reality-testing and identity-checking;
- not-knowing;
- 'moral' judging.

In Essay 1 (p. 40), we saw that reflection has the specific job of enhancing reality-testing to support the members of staff against the sense of failure likely to arise from their unconscious expectations of themselves. It has an important part to play in tackling the stereotype of the all-healthy and all-wise staff.

However, there is a paradox if one of the crucial ways in which the carer can succeed is to get to a level of not-knowing. Reflection on not-knowing is an uncommon competence, or at least does not normally reside within the area of general competence. Yet work with psychosis is not normal work. It is not to be confused with any general kind of work. It is work with the incomprehensible.

Moreover, if we put the humility of not-knowing alongside the identity of the all-wise carer, we have a sobering check on the identity distortion that we are prone to suffer unwittingly in psychiatric care. Reflection on the lack of meaning will very likely have an effect on the drive for perfect cures and the omnipotent level of super-ego demand.

Another area of work in the reflective mode is about the 'moral' qualities of patients and staff (see Barham 1984). To like or to hate each other is an important aspect of human relating, and insofar as it is put on hold when working with schizophrenic patients it depersonalises them – and to an extent the staff. To like or dislike is a judgement upon the person's worth, and is gauged on her acts. Her actions or behaviour, which are liked or disliked, can and will be adjudged by her carers. As Barrett (Essay 1, 'Meaninglessness and understanding', p. 16) has described, the final stage of treatment of a schizophrenic is to bring her back as a moral being. Barrett's account described an important step-like process that a psychotic patient undergoes after admission to a psychiatric hospital (Barrett 1996; see Essay 1). Each step requires a different personal approach from the staff team, starting with a most neutral and objective attitude and finishing with a much more personally involved and authentic relating. Each step requires the professional carer to adopt a changing pattern of personal and emotional attitudes. In the later phase, when patients are accepted once again as agents with volition, there is a neglect of any formal support for that personal relating. That phase requires emotional and moral evaluation from us. Professionals normally avoid moral judgements about their patients, but in so doing they inevitably and counter-intuitively denude patients of personhood. Of course mental health workers *do* actually show such moral attitudes. Whether we accept it or not, we like/dislike, approve/disapprove of patients and their use of us. Such judgements are plentiful in tea-room conversations when staff relax, where they cannot be called to account. This gives our humanity an off-duty quality, yet these *sotto voce* evaluations are essential, because they endow the patient with agency and personhood. Such judgemental attitudes hold patients responsible for how they are and what they do, and thus at the right moment restore humanity and personhood – albeit a painful self-awareness.

In fact not all schizophrenic patients do make it back. Nor are all staff sufficiently supported in this phase. Some patients become trapped at this stage, where at best they can remain a 'worked-up' case with a treatment programme, but do not emerge into personhood again. Such casualties are then regarded as the chronic or intractable cases. However, when all goes well the patient is returned to being a person, 'given back', as it were, her own agency, and rescued from the category of a 'case'.

In this mode, there is a tendency to give moral worth to the person of the patient. Certainly it is of considerable distress to be disliked as a person – and unwittingly seductive to be liked as a person. It is important for staff to recognise this as a personal reaction, which on reflection needs unpacking in detail. Reflection needs to unpack the dislike of the person in terms of what he actually does, or the likeable things he does. If we stick simply with disliking him as a person, or liking him as a person, we have moved to a personal relationship, and implicitly away from the professional. We need to reflect on his actual behaviour that gives rise to sweeping judgements about liking or disliking him as a person. Our emotional reactions to the specific behaviours contribute to our relation to his whole existential being, and thus contribute to confirming it. However, our role as psychiatric professionals is to confirm his being through his responsibility for himself. That means acknowledging what he does, and liking that or not as the case may be.

It is of course not so easy to stick simply to what the patient does. He does strange things to us; he intrudes through his actions and behaviour into our minds and our beings. That active interaction is his *modus operandi*, his means of communication once he has abandoned ordinary symbols. Therefore, carers can be particularly provoked to react inappropriately to him as a person, when the impact is on our emotional being as persons. This is why a process of reflection, and its support by each other, and if necessary an external consultant to keep the reflection fresh and honest, are important. Perhaps in the process of reflection with each other it could be a specified strategy to probe reactions to patients in terms of what exactly they have done, said or indicated that gives rise to the positive or negative response in the carer.

An unspoken contract develops between patient and staff, which seems particularly intimate. It goes back to the question with which we started – who is going to suffer the insanity? The psychotic patient completely confounds the assumption that he will. Instead, his carers feel the responsibility that he will not suffer. His carers suffer the awful knowledge of meaninglessness, which he will not. The most abbreviated summary of the message of this book is that we are all in the same boat. Psychologically we have to suffer something of our patient's suffering. We have to know psychosis in the way he knows it. This obliges us to start our work with the acceptance that we have our own psychology, the psychology of care, and we need to study it. And inevitably we need to study it inside ourselves as well as in books like this one.

I am concluding this book with these first steps in the reflective process that we need to engage in. It is 'inner' work, emotional labour, that our patients need of us. Reflection, insofar as it is possible, has three areas of operation in the mind of carers:

- reality of small successes;
- not-knowing;
- moral judgement.

When of value, reflection allows a patient to find his own space, however small, to begin such reflection upon himself. At first, this seems to begin when the carer joins the patient in some shared experience of the patient, probably in sharing the experience of meaninglessness.

This programme of reflection is not intended to be definitive, but to be an initial exploration of what is needed. It will in any case be a unique process of reflection arising from the unique needs and character of each person. Variation allows us to enhance our own work through others' ways of looking at things. It is not offered as a command to perfection, but merely as a tentative signpost towards which we might aspire. There is nothing that can substitute for authentic responding; the slide into ritualisation, as indicated in the Essay 3 ('Risks and rituals', p. 151), is a short cut that leads us into a diversion away from the painful slog of the work.

References

Abraham, K. (1911) Notes on the psychoanalytical investigation and treatment of manic-depressive insanity and allied conditions. In K. Abraham, *Selected Papers on Psychoanalysis*. London: Hogarth, 1927.

Abraham, K. (1924) A short study of the development of the libido viewed in the light of mental disorders. In K. Abraham (1927) *Selected Papers on Psychoanalysis*. London: Hogarth Press.

Ackerman, N. (1958) *The Psychodynamics of Family Life: Diagnosis and Treatment of Family Relationships*. New York: Basic Books.

Alanen, Y.O., Lehtinen, K., Räkköläinen, V. and Aaltonen, J. (1991) Need-adapted treatment of new schizophrenic patients; experiences and results of the Turku project. *Acta Psychiatrica Scandinavia* **83**: 363–372.

American Psychiatric Association (1994) *Diagnostic Criteria fron DSM-IV*. Washington, DC: APA.

Atwood, G. and Stolorow, R. (1984) *Structures of Subjectivity*. Hillside, NJ: Analytic Press.

Balint, M. (1957) *The Doctor, His Patient and the Illness*. London: Tavistock.

Barham, P. (1984) *Schizophrenia and Human Value*. Oxford: Blackwell.

Barnes, E., Griffiths, P., Ord, J. and Wells, D. (1998) *Face to Face with Distress: The Professional Use of Self in Psychosocial Care*. Oxford: Butterworth-Heinemann.

Barrett, Rob (1996) *The Psychiatric Team and the Social Definition of Schizophrenia*. Cambridge: Cambridge University Press.

Bateman, A. and Fonagy, P. (1999) Effectiveness of partial hospitalization in the treatment of Borderline Personality Disorder: a randomised controlled trial. *American Journal of Psychiatry* **156**: 1563.

Bateman, A. and Fonagy, P. (2001) Treatment of Borderline Personality Disorder with a psychoanalytically oriented partial hospitalization: an 18 month follow up. *American Journal of Psychiatry* **158**: 36–42.

Bateson, G., Jackson, D., Haley, J. and Weakland, J. (1956) Toward a theory of schizophrenia. *Behavioral Science* **1**: 251–264.

Beckett, S. (1935) Cited by Lawrence Harvey in interview with Jim Knowlson, 1962, and quoted in Knowlson (1996), p. 209.

Berke, J. (1979) *I Haven't Had to Go Mad Here*. London: Penguin.

Berke, J.H., Fagan, M., Mak-Pearce, G. and Pierides-Müller, S. (eds) (2001) *Beyond Madness: Psychosocial Interventions in Psychosis*. London: Jessica Kingsley.

Bhaskar, R. (1979) *The Possibility of Naturalism: A Philosophical Critique of the Contemporary Human Sciences*. London: Routledge.

Bion, W.R. (1954) Notes on the theory of schizophrenia. *International Journal of Psychoanalysis* **35**: 113–118. Expanded as 'Language and the schizophrenic' in M. Klein, P. Heimann and R. Money-Kyrle (eds) (1955) *New Directions in Psychoanalysis*, London: Tavistock. Republished in W.R. Bion (1967) *Second Thoughts*, London: Heinemann.

Bion, W.R. (1957) Differentiation of the psychotic form the non-psychotic parts of the ego. *International Journal of Psychoanalysis* **38**: 266–275. Republished in W.R. Bion (1967) *Second Thoughts*, London: Heinemann; and in E. Bott Spillius (1988) *Melanie Klein Today*. Vol. 1, London: Routledge.

Bion, W.R. (1959) Attacks on linking. *International Journal of Psychoanalysis* **40**: 308–315. Republished in W.R. Bion (1967) *Second Thoughts*, London: Heinemann; and in E. Bott Spillius (1988) *Melanie Klein Today*, Vol. 1, London: Routledge.

Bion, W.R. (1961) *Experiences in Groups*. London: Tavistock.

Bion, W.R. (1962a) A theory of thinking. *International Journal of Psychoanalysis* **43**: 306–310. Republished in W.R. Bion (1967) *Second Thoughts*, London: Heinemann; and in E. Bott Spillius (1988) *Melanie Klein Today*, Vol. 1, London: Routledge.

Bion, W.R. (1962b) *Learning from Experience*. London: Heinemann.

Bleuler, E. (1911/1955) *Dementia Praecox or the Group of Schizophrenias*. London: Allen and Unwin.

Bowlby, J. (1969) *Attachment and Loss*. London: Hogarth.

Brenman-Pick, I. (1985) Working through in the countertransference. *International Journal of Psycho-Analysis* **66**: 157–166. In E. Bott Spillius (1988), *Melanie Klein Today*. London: Routledge.

Breuer, J. and Freud, S. (1895) The psychical mechanism of hysterical phenomena: preliminary communication. In *Studies in Hysteria. The Standard Edition of the Complete Psychological Works of Sigmund Freud*, Vol. 2. London: Hogarth.

Butler, S. (1880) *Unconscious Memory*. London: Jonathan Cape.

Chiesa, M. and Fonagy, P. (2000) Cassel personality disorder study: methodology and treatment effects. *British Journal of Psychiatry* **176**: 485–491.

Chiesa, M., Fonagy, P., Holmes, J., Drahorad, C. and Harrison-Hall, A. (2002) Health service use costs by personality disorder following specialist and non-specialist treatment: a comparative study. *Journal of Personality Disorders* **16**: 160–173.

Clark, D. (1964) *Administrative Therapy*. London: Tavistock.

Clarke, S. (2003) Social theory, psychoanalysis, and racism. New York: Palgrave.

Conran, M. (1985) The patient in hospital. *Psychoanalytic Psychotherapy* **1**: 31–43.

Conran, M. (1999) Sorrow, vulnerability and madness. In P. Williams (ed.) *Psychosis (Madness)*. London: Institute of Psychoanalysis.

Craib, I. (1998) *Experiencing Identity*. London: Sage.

Cullberg, J. (2001) 'The parachute project': first episode psychosis – background and treatment. In P. Williams (ed.) *A Language for Psychosis*. London: Whurr.

Davies, R. (1996) The interdisciplinary network and the internal world of the offender. In C. Cordess and M. Cox (eds) *Forensic Psychotherapy*, Vol. 2. London: Jessica Kingsley.

Day, L. and Pringle, P. (2001) *Reflective Enquiry into Therapeutic Institutions*. London: Karnac.

Deleuze, G. and Guatari, F. (1972) *L'Anti-Oedipe: Capitalisme et Schizophrénie*. Paris: Minuit. English translation (1983), *Anti-Oedipus: Capitalism and Schizophrenia*. London: Athlone.

de Vries, K. (ed.) (1991) *Organisations on the Couch*. San Francisco: Jossey-Bass.

Donald, A. (1998) The worlds we live in. In T. Greenhalgh and B. Hurwitz (eds) *Narrative Based Medicine: Dialogue and Discourse in Clinical Practice*. London: BMJ Books.

Donati, Flavia (1989) Madness and morale. *British Journal of Psychotherapy* **5**: 317–329. Republished in R.D. Hinshelwood and W. Skogstad (eds) (2000) *Observing Organisations*. London: Routledge.

Dupont, J. (1988) Ferenczi's 'madness'. *Contemporary Psychoanalysis* **24**: 250–261.

Eissler, K. 1951 Remarks on the psychoanalysis of schizophrenia. *International Journal of Psychoanalysis* **32**: 139–156.

Ellenberger, H.F. (1974) *The Discovery of the Unconscious. The History and Evolution of Dynamic Psychiatry*. New York: Basic Books.

Ellwood, J. (1995) *Psychosis: Understanding and Treatment*. London: Jessica Kingsley.

Emde, R. and Fonagy, P. (1997) An emerging culture for psychoanalytic research? *International Journal of Psychoanalysis* **78**: 643–651.

Federn, P. (1934) The analysis of psychotics. *International Journal of Psychoanalysis* **15**: 209–215.

Figlio, K. (1982) How does illness mediate social relations? Workmen's compensation and medical-legal practices, 1890–1940. In A. Treacher and P. Wright (eds), *The Problem of Medical Knowledge: Examining the*

Social Construction of Medicine. Edinburgh: Edinburgh University Press, pp. 174–224.

Fineman, S. (1993) *Emotion in Organisations*. London: Sage.

Fonagy, P. (1999) Evidence-based medicine and its justifications. In M. Leuzinger-Bohleber and M. Target (eds) *Outcomes of Psychoanalytic Treatment*. London: Whurr.

Foster, A. (1998) Psychotic processes and community care. In A. Foster and V. Roberts (eds) *Managing Mental Health in the Community: Chaos and Containment in Community Care*. London: Routledge.

Foster, A. and Roberts, V. (eds) (1998) *Managing Mental Health in the Community: Chaos and Containment*. London: Routledge.

Foucault, M. (1967) *Madness and Civilisation*. London: Tavistock.

Frame, J. (1962) *Faces in the Water*. London: W.H. Allen.

Freud, S. (1900) The interpretation of dreams. *The Standard Edition of the Complete Psychological Works of Sigmund Freud*, Vols 4 and 5. London: Hogarth Press.

Freud, S. (1905) Fragment of an analysis of a case of hysteria. *The Standard Edition of the Complete Psychological Works of Sigmund Freud*, Vol. 7, pp. 7–122. London: Hogarth Press.

Freud, S. (1909a) Analysis of a phobia in a five-year-old boy. *The Standard Edition of the Complete Psychological Works of Sigmund Freud*, Vol. 10. London: Hogarth Press.

Freud, S. (1909b) Notes upon a case of obsessional neurosis. *The Standard Edition of the Complete Psychological Works of Sigmund Freud*, Vol. 10. London: Hogarth Press.

Freud, S. (1911a) Psycho-analytic notes on an autobiographical account of a case of paranoia. *Standard Edition of the Complete Psychological Works of Sigmund Freud*, Vol. 12. London: Hogarth Press.

Freud, S. (1911b) Formulations regarding the two principles of mental functioning. *Standard Edition of the Complete Psychological Works of Sigmund Freud*, Vol. 12. London: Hogarth Press.

Freud, S. (1914) On narcissism. *The Standard Edition of the Complete Psychological Works of Sigmund Freud*, Vol. 14, pp. 73–102. London: Hogarth Press.

Freud, S. (1915) The unconscious. *The Standard Edition of the Complete Psychological Works of Sigmund Freud*, Vol. 10, p. 155. London: Hogarth Press.

Freud, S. (1917a) Mourning and melancholia. *The Standard Edition of the Complete Psychological Works of Sigmund Freud*, Vol. 14. London: Hogarth Press.

Freud, S. (1917b) Metapsychological supplement to dreams. *The Standard Edition of the Complete Psychological Works of Sigmund Freud*, Vol. 14. London: Hogarth Press.

Freud, S. (1917c) Introductory lecture 16: Psychoanalysis and psychiatry.

The Standard Edition of the Complete Psychological Works of Sigmund Freud, Vol. 16. London: Hogarth Press.

Freud, S. (1923) The ego and the id. *The Standard Edition of the Complete Psychological Works of Sigmund Freud*, Vol. 19, pp. 12–66. London: Hogarth Press.

Freud, S. (1924a) Neurosis and psychosis. *The Standard Edition of the Complete Psychological Works of Sigmund Freud*, Vol. 19, p. 149. London: Hogarth Press.

Freud, S. (1924b) The loss of reality in neurosis and psychosis. *The Standard Edition of the Complete Psychological Works of Sigmund Freud*, Vol. 19, pp. 183–187. London: Hogarth Press.

Freud, S. (1940) An outline of psychoanalysis. *The Standard Edition of the Complete Psychological Works of Sigmund Freud*, Vol. 23. London: Hogarth Press.

Fromm-Reichman, F. (1939) Transference problems in schizophrenics. *Psychoanalytic Quarterly* **8**: 412–426.

Goffman, E. (1961) *Asylums*. London: Penguin.

Green, H. (1964) *I Never Promised You a Rose Garden*. New York: New American Library.

Greenhalgh, T. (1998) Narrative based medicine in an evidence based world. In T. Greenhalgh and B. Hurwitz (eds) *Narrative Based Medicine: Dialogue and Discourse in Clinical Practice*. London: BMJ Books.

Greenhalgh, T. and Hurwitz, B. (1998) Why study narrative? In T. Greenhalgh and Brian H. (eds) *Narrative Based Medicine: Dialogue and Discourse in Clinical Practice*. London: BMJ Books.

Griffiths, P. (1997) *Psychosocial Practice within a Residential Setting*. London: Karnac.

Griffiths, P. and Hinshelwood, R.D. (1997) Actions speak louder than words. In P. Griffiths, *Psychosocial Practice within a Residential Setting*. London: Karnac.

Griffiths, P. and Hinshelwood, R.D. 2001 Enquiring into a culture of enquiry. In L. Day and Pam P. (eds) *Reflective Enquiry into Therapeutic Institutions*. London: Karnac.

Griffiths, R. (1983) *NHS Management Inquiry*. London: Department of Health & Social Security.

Grotstein, J. (2001) A rationale for psychoanalytically informed psychotherapy of schizophrenia and other psychoses; towards the concept of 'rehabilitative psychoanalysis'. In P. Williams (ed.) *A Language for Psychosis*. London: Whurr.

Guntrip, H. (1967) The concept of psychodynamic science. *International Journal of Psychoanalysis* **38**: 32–43.

Habermas, J. (1971) *Knowledge and Human Interests*. Boston: Beacon Press.

Hacking, I. (1999) *The Social Construction of What?* Cambridge, MA: Harvard University Press.

Hampe, M. (2000) Pluralismus der Wissenschaften und die Einheit der Vernunft. In M. Hame (ed.) *Die Erfahrungen, die wir machen, widersprechen den Erfahringen, die wir haben: Formen der Erfahrungen in den Wissenschaften*. Berlin: Dunker und Humblot.

Harlow, H.F. (1961) The development of affectional patterns in infant monkeys. In B.M. Foss (ed.) *Determinants of Infant Behaviour*, Vol. 1. London: Methuen.

Heimann, P. (1942) A contribution to the problem of sublimation and its relation to processes of internalisation. *International Journal of Psychoanalysis* **23**: 8–17.

Heimann, P. (1950) On countertransference. *International Journal of Psychoanalysis* **31**: 81–84.

Hinshelwood, R.D. (1979) Demoralisation and the hospital community. *Group Analysis* **12**, 84–93. Republished in R.D. Hinshelwood (2001) *Thinking about Institutions*. London: Jessica Kingsley.

Hinshelwood, R.D. (1983) Projective identification and Marx's concept of man. *International Review of Psychoanalysis* **16**: 221–226.

Hinshelwood, R.D. (1987a) *What Happens in Groups: Psychoanalysis, the Individual and the Community*. London: Free Association Books.

Hinshelwood, R.D. (1987b) The psychotherapist's role in a large mental institution. *Psychoanalytic Psychotherapy* **2**: 207–215.

Hinshelwood, R.D. (1987c) Social dynamics and individual symptoms. *International Journal of Therapeutic Communities* **8**: 265.

Hinshelwood, R.D. (1989a) Social possession of identity. In B. Richards (ed.) *Crises of the Self*. London: Free Association Books.

Hinshelwood, R.D. (1989b) Communication flow in the matrix. *Group Analysis* **22**: 261–269.

Hinshelwood, R.D. (1993) Locked in role: a psychotherapist within the social defence system of a prison. *Journal of Forensic Psychiatry* **4**: 427–440.

Hinshelwood, R.D. (1994a) Integrity of the person and the day hospital: evidence from a therapeutic community. *International Journal of Therapeutic Communities* **15**: 29–38.

Hinshelwood, R.D. (1994b) The relevance of psychotherapy, *Psycho-Analytic Psychotherapy* **8**: 283–294.

Hinshelwood, R.D. (1997) *Therapy or Coercion: Does Psychoanalysis Differ from Brainwashing?* London: Karnac.

Hinshelwood, R.D. (1998) Creatures of each other: some historical considerations of responsibility and care and some present undercurrents. In A. Foster and V.Z. Roberts (eds) *Managing Mental Health in the Community: Chaos and Containment*. London: Routledge.

Hinshelwood, R.D. (1999) The difficult patient: the role of 'scientific' psychiatry in understanding patients with chronic schizophrenia or severe personality disorder. *British Journal of Psychiatry* **174**: 187–190.

Hinshelwood, R.D. (2000) Alienation: social relations and therapeutic relations. *Psychoanalytic Studies* **2**: 21–30.

Hinshelwood, R.D. (2001) *Thinking about Institutions*. London: Jessica Kingsley.

Hinshelwood, R.D. (2002) Symptoms or relationships. *British Medical Journal* **324**: 292–293.

Hinshelwood, R.D. (2003) Group mentality and 'having a mind'. In M. Pines and B. Lipgar (eds) *Building on Bion*, Vol. 1. London: Jessica Kingsley.

Hinshelwood, R.D. and Skogstad, W. (eds) (2000) *Observing Organisations*. London: Routledge.

Hobson, P., Patrick, M. and Valentine, J.D. (1998) Objectivity in psychoanalytic judgments. *British Journal of Psychiatry* **173**: 172–177.

Hochschild, A. (1983) *The Managed Heart*. Berkeley: University of California Press.

Holland, E. (1999) *Deleuze and Guattari's Anti-Oedipus: Introduction to Schizoanalysis*. London: Routledge.

Holmes, J. (1993) *John Bowlby and Attachment Theory*. London: Routledge.

Holmes, J. (2002) All you need is cognitive therapy. *British Medical Journal* **324**: 288–290.

Hopfl, H. and Linstead, S. (1993) Passion and performance: suffering and the carrying of organisational roles. In S. Fineman (ed.) *Emotion in Organisations*. London: Sage.

Horwitz, A. (2002) *Creating Mental Illness*. Chicago: University of Chicago Press.

Isaacs, S. (1948) The nature and function of phantasy. *International Journal of Psychoanalysis* **29**: 73–97. Republished in Klein, M., Heimann, P., Isaacs, S. and Riviere, J. (1952) *New Directions in Psychoanalysis*. London: Hogarth Press.

Jackson, M. (1993) Manic-depressive psychosis: psychopathology and individual psychotherapy within a psychodynamic milieu. *Psychoanalytic Psychotherapy* **7**: 103–133.

Jackson, M. (2001) *Weathering the Storms*. London: Karnac.

Jackson, M. and Williams, P. (1994) *Unimaginable Storms*. London: Karnac.

Janet, P. (1892) *États mental des hystériques*. Paris: J. Rueff.

Jaques, E. (1955) Social systems as a defence against persecutory and depressive anxiety. In M. Klein, P. Heimann and R.E. Money-Kyrle (eds) *New Directions in Psychoanalysis*. London: Tavistock. Republished in E. Trist and H. Murray (eds) (1990) *The Social Engagement of Social Science*, Vol. 1: *The Socio-Psychological Perspective*. London: Free Association Books, pp. 420–438.

Jones, E. (1929) Psychoanalysis and psychiatry. In E. Jones (1948) *Papers on Psychoanalysis*. London: Bailliere, Tindall and Cox.

Jung, C. (1906) The psychological significance of the association experiment.

The Collected Works of C.G. Jung, Vol. 2. Princeton, NJ: Princeton University Press, 1973.

Kanner, L. (1943) Autistic disturbances of affective contact. *Nervous Child* **2**: 217–250.

Katan, M. (1954) The importance of the non-psychotic part of the personality in schizophrenia. *International Journal of Psychoanalysis* **35**: 119–128.

Kesey, K. (1962) *One Flew over the Cuckoo's Nest*. New York: Viking.

Klein, M. (1930) The importance of symbol formation in the development of the ego. In *The Writings of Melanie Klein*, Vol. 1, pp. 219–232. London: Hogarth Press.

Klein, M. (1935) A contribution to the psychogenesis of manic-depressive states. *International Journal of Psychoanalysis* **16**: 145–174.

Klein, M. (1940) Mourning and its relation to manic-depressive states. *International Journal of Psychoanalysis* **21**: 125–153.

Klein, M. (1946) Notes on some schizoid mechanisms. In *The Writings of Melanie Klein*, Vol. 3: 1–24. London: Hogarth Press.

Klein, M. (1955) On identification. In *The Writings of Melanie Klein*, Vol. 3, pp. 141–175. London: Hogarth Press.

Kleinman, A. (1988) *The Illness Narratives*. New York: Basic Books.

Knowlson, J. (1996) *Damned to Fame: The Life of Samuel Beckett*. London: Bloomsbury.

Kraepelin, E. (1905) *Psychiatrie: Ein Lehrbuch*. Leipzig: Barth Verlag. Translated in part as Kraepelin, E. (1919) *Dementia Praecox and Paraphrenia*. Edinburgh: Livingstone.

Lacan, J. (1955–1956/1981) *Le Séminaire. Livre III. Les psychoses*. Paris: Seuil.

Lacan, J. (1949) Le Stade du Mirror comme formateur de la fonction du Je. In J. Lacan (1966) *Écrits*. Paris: Seuil. English translation, as 'The mirror stage as formative of the function of the I', in J. Lacan (1977) *Écrits: A Selection*. London: Tavistock.

Laing, R.D. (1960) *The Divided Self*. London: Tavistock.

Laing, R.D. (1967) *The Politics of Experience*. London: Penguin.

Laing, R.D. and Esterson, A. (1964) *Sanity, Madness and the Family*. London: Tavistock.

Leff, J. (1997) *Care in the Community: Illusion or Reality?* Chichester: Wiley.

Leuzinger-Bohleber, M. (2002) Introductory remarks. In M. Leuzinger-Bohleber and M. Target (eds) *Outcomes of Psychoanalytic Treatment*. London: Whurr.

Levenson, E. (1992) Harry Stack Sullivan: from interpersonal psychiatry to interpersonal psychoanalysis. *Contemporary Psychoanalysis* **28**: 450–466.

Lidz, T. (1963) *The Family and Human Adaptation*. London: Hogarth Press.

Linstead, S. and Hopfl, H. (2000) *The Aesthetics of Organisations*. London: Sage.

Lucas, R. (1993) The psychotic wavelength. *Psychoanalytic Psychotherapy* **7**: 15–24.

Lucas, R. (1998) Why the cycle in a cyclical psychosis? An analytic understating of the recurrent manic-depressive psychosis. *Psychoanalytic Psychotherapy* **6**: 193–212.

Lucas, R. (2003) The relationship between psychoanalysis and schizophrenia. *International Journal of Psychoanalysis* **84**: 3–15.

Macalpine, I. and Hunter, R.A. (1955) Introduction to *Memoirs of my Nervous Illness/Daniel Paul Schreber*. London: Dawson.

Mace, C., Moorey, S. and Roberts, B. (eds) (2001) *Evidence in the Psychological Therapies*. London: Routledge.

McPherson, S., Richardson, P. and Leroux, P. (2003) (eds) *Clinical Effectiveness in Psychotherapy and Mental Health*. London: Karnac.

Main, T.H. (1946) The hospital as a therapeutic institution. *Bulletin of the Menninger Clinic* **10**: 66–70.

Main, T. (1957) The ailment. *British Journal of Medical Psychology* **30**: 129–145. Republished in T.F. Main (1989) *The Ailment and Other Psychoanalytic Essays*. London: Free Association Books.

Main, T.F. (1967) Knowledge, learning and freedom from thought. *Australian and New Zealand Journal of Psychiatry* **1**: 64–71. Republished in *Psychoanalytic Psychotherapy* (1990) **15**: 59–74.

Main, T.F. (1975) Some psychodynamics of large groups. In L. Kreeger (ed.) *The Large Group*. London: Constable. Republished in Main, T.F. (1989) *The Ailment and Other Psychoanalytic Essays*. London: Free Association Books.

Martin, D. (1955) Institutionalisation. *Lancet*, no. **2**: 1188–1190.

Martinez-Hernaez, Angel (2000) *What's Behind the Symptom? On Psychiatric Observation and Anthropological Understanding*. New York: Routledge.

Marx, Karl (1844) *1844 Economic and Philosophical Manuscripts*. London: Penguin.

Meltzer, D. (1963) A contribution to the metapsychology of cyclothymic states. *International Journal of Psychoanalysis* **44**: 83–96.

Meltzer, D. (1978) A note on Bion's concept of 'Reversal of alpha-function'. In D. Metzer, *The Kleinian Development, Part III*. Strath Tay, Perthshire: Clunie Press.

Menzies, I. (1959) A case study in the functioning of social systems as a defence against anxiety. *Human Relations* **13**: 95–121. Republished in I. Menzies (1988) *Containing Anxiety in Institutions*. London: Free Association Books.

Menzies, I. (1979) Staff support systems: task and antitask in adolescent institutions. In R.D. Hinshelwood and N. Manning, *Therapeutic Communities: Reflections and Progress*. London: Routledge and Kegan Paul. Republished in I. Menzies (1988) *Containing Anxiety in Institutions*. London: Free Association Books.

Miller, E. and Gwynne, G.V. (1972) *A Life Apart*. London: Tavistock.

Miller, E.J. and Rice A.K. (1967) *Systems of Organisation*. London: Tavistock.

Myers, F. (1903) *Human Personality and its Survival of Death*. London: Longmans, Green.

Norton, K. (1992) A culture of enquiry: its preservation or loss. *Therapeutic Communities* **13**: 3–25.

Nunberg, H. (1931) The synthetic function of the ego. *International Journal of Psycho-Analysis*, **12**: 123–140.

Nunberg, H. (1950) A commentary on Freud's 'An outline of psychoanalysis'. *Psychoanalytic Quarterly* **19**: 227–250.

Obholzer, A. and Roberts, V. (1994) *The Unconscious at Work*. London: Routledge.

Platt, R. (1965) Thoughts on teaching medicine. *British Medical Journal*, no. **2**: 551–552.

Racker, H. (1968) *Transference and Countertransference*. London: Hogarth.

Rado, S. (1928) An anxious mother: a contribution to the analysis of the ego. *International Journal of Psychoanalysis* **9**: 219–226.

Read, S. (1989) *Only for a Fortnight: My Life in a Locked Ward*. London: Bloomsbury.

Reilly, S. (1997) Psychoanalytic and psychodynamic perspectives to psychosis: an overview. In C. Mace and F. Margison, *Psychotherapy of Psychosis*. London: Gaskell.

Renik, O. (1993) Analytic interaction: conceptualizing technique in light of the analyst's irreducible subjectivity. *Psychoanalytic Quarterly* **62**: 553–571.

Rey, H. (1994) That which patients bring to analysis. *International Journal of Psychoanalysis* **68**: 457–470.

Riccoeur, P. (1981) *Hermeneutics and the Human Sciences*. Cambridge: Cambridge University Press.

Richardson, P. (2001) Evidence-based practice and the psychodynamic psychotherapies. In C. Mace, S. Moorey and B. Roberts (eds) *Evidence in the Psychological Therapies*. London: Routledge.

Rorty, R. (1979) *Philosophy and the Mirror of Nature*. Princeton, NJ: Princeton University Press.

Rosen, J. (1947) The treatment of schizophrenic psychosis by direct analytic therapy. *Psychiatric Quarterly* **21**: 3–17, 117–119.

Rosenberg, S.D. (1970) Hospital culture as a collective defence. *Psychiatry* **33**: 21–38.

Rosenfeld, H. (1952) Notes on the psycho-analysis of the super-ego conflict of an acute schizophrenic patient. *International Journal of Psychoanalysis* **33**: 111–131. Republished in H. Rosenfeld (1965) *Psychotic States*, London: Hogarth; and in E. Bott Spillius (1988) *Melanie Klein Today*, Vol. 1, London: Routledge.

Rosenfeld, H. (1964) On the psychopathology of narcissism: a clinical approach. *International Journal of Psychoanalysis* **45**: 332–337.

Rosenfeld, H. (1965) *Psychotic States*. London: Hogarth Press.

Rosenfeld, H. (1971) A clinical approach to the psychoanalytic theory of the life and death instincts: an investigation into the aggressive aspects of narcissism. *International Journal of Psychoanalysis* **52**: 169–178. Republished in E. Bott Spillius (1988) *Melanie Klein Today*, Vol. 1. London: Routledge.

Roth, A. and Fonagy, P. (1996) *What Works for Whom?* New York: Guilford.

Samuels, A. (1986) *A Critical Dictionary of Jungian Analysis*. London: Routledge and Kegan Paul.

Samuels, A. (1989) *Psychopathology: Contemporary Jungian Perspectives*. London: Karnac.

Schatzman, M. (1973) *Soul Murder: Persecution in the Family*. London: Allen Lane.

Schneider, K. (1959) *Clinical Psychopathology*. New York: Grune and Stratton.

Schreber, D.G.M. (1858) *Kallipoedie oder Erziehung zur Schönheit durch naturgetreu und gleichmässige Förderung normaler Körperbildung*. Leipzig: F. Fleischer.

Schreber, D.P. (1903) *Denkwürdigkeiten eines Nervenkranken*. English translation: In I. Macalpine and R.A. Hunter (trans and eds) (1955) *Memoirs of my Nervous Illness*. London: Dawson.

Scruton, R. (1983) *A Dictionary of Political Thought*. London: Pan.

Scull, A. (1977) *Decarceration*. Cambridge: Polity Press.

Searles, H. (1979) *Countertransference and Related Subjects*. New York: International Universities Press.

Sechehaye, M. (1951) *Autobiography of a Schizophrenic Girl*. New York: Grune and Stratton.

Segal, H. (1950) Some aspects of the analysis of a schizophrenic. *International Journal of Psychoanalysis* **31**: 268–278. Republished in *The Works of Hanna Segal* (1981), London: Free Association Books; and in E. Bott Spillius (1988) *Melanie Klein Today*, Vol. 1, London: Routledge.

Segal, H. (1957) Notes on symbol formation. *International Journal of Psychoanalysis* **38**: 391–397. Republished in *The Works of Hanna Segal* (1981), London: Free Association Books; and in E. Bott Spillius (1988) *Melanie Klein Today*, Vol. 1, London: Routledge.

Shengold, L. (1989) *Soul Murder. The Effects of Childhood Abuse and Deprivation*. New Haven, CT: Yale University Press.

Sinason, M. (1993) Who is the mad voice inside? *Psychoanalytic Psychotherapy* **7**: 207–221.

Sohn, L. (1995) Unprovoked assaults – making sense of apparently random violence. *International Journal of Psychoanalysis* **76**: 565–575.

Sohn, L. (1999) Psychosis and violence. In P. Williams (ed.) *Psychosis (Madness)*. London: Institute of Psychoanalysis.
Sontag, S. (1983) *Illness as Metaphor*. London: Penguin.
Spillius, E. Bott (1976) Hospital and society. *British Journal of Medical Psychology* **49**: 97–140. Abridged version published as 'Asylum and society' in E. Trist and H. Murray (eds) 1990 *The Social Engagement of Social Science*, Vol. 1: *The Socio-Psychological Perspective*. London: Free Association Books.
Stanton, A.H. and Schwartz, H.S. (1954) *The Mental Hospital*, New York: Basic Books.
Stapley, L. (1996) *The Personality of the Organisation*. London: Free Association Books.
Steiner, J. (1993) *Psychic Retreats*. London: Hogarth Press.
Stokes, J. (1994) The unconscious at work in groups and teams. In A. Obholzer and V. Roberts (eds) *The Unconscious at Work*. London: Routledge.
Sullivan, H.S. (1962) *Schizophrenia as a Human Process*. New York: W.W. Norton.
Taylor, F. (1911) *The Principles of Scientific Management*. New York: Harper Bros.
Theodosius, C. (2003) *Developing the sociology of emotion and emotional labour: a case study of nurses*. PhD Thesis, University of Essex.
Thompson, C. (1978) Sullivan and psychoanalysis. *Contemporary Psychoanalysis* **14**: 488–501.
Trist, E. (1950/1990) Culture as a psychosocial process. In E. Trist and H. Murray (eds) *The Social Engagement of Social Science*, Vol. 1: *The Socio-Psychological Perspective*. London: Free Association Books.
Vaughn, C. and Leff, J. (1976) The measurement of expressed emotion in the families of psychiatric patients. *British Journal of Social and Clinical Psychology* **15**: 157–165.
Wallerstein, R. (2000) Psychoanalytic research: where do we disagree? In J. Sandler, A.M. Sandler and R. Davies (eds) *Clinical and Observational Psychoanalytic Research*. London: Karnac.
Weber, M. (1954) *Economy and Society*. Cambridge, MA: Harvard University Press.
Wexler, M. (1965) Working through in the therapy of schizophrenia. *International Journal of Psychoanalysis* **46**: 279–286.
Wexler, M. (1971) Schizophrenia: conflict and deficiency. *Psychoanalytic Quarterly* **40**: 83–99.
Whitehead, A. and Russell, B. (1910) *Principia Mathematica*. Cambridge: Cambridge University Press.
Whyte, L. (1978) *The Unconscious before Freud*. London: Julian Friedman.
Williams, P. (2001) *A Language for Psychosis*. London: Whurr.

Williams, R. (1958) *Culture and Society 1780–1950*. London: Chatto & Windus.

Willick, M.S. (2001) Psychoanalysis and schizophrenia: a cautionary tale. *Journal of the American Psychoanalytic Association* **9**: 27–56.

Winnicott, D. (1949) Hate in the countertransference. *International Journal of Psychoanalysis* **30**: 69–74. Republished in D. Winnicott (1958) *Through Paediatrics to Psychoanalysis*. London: Tavistock.

Winnicott, D. (1960) The theory of the parent-infant relationship. *International Journal of Psychoanalysis* **41**: 585–595. Republished in D. Winnicott (1965) *The Maturational Processes and the Facilitating Environment*. London: Hogarth Press.

Winnicott, D. (1967) Mirror-role of mother and family in child development. In P. Lomas (ed.) *The Predicament of the Family*. London: Hogarth Press.

Index